DATE DUE

MEDICAL CARE

of

PATIENTS WITH
HIV INFECTION

12th Edition

The Johns Hopkins Hospital 2005-6 Guide to

MEDICAL CARE

of

PATIENTS WITH HIV INFECTION

12th Edition

John G. Bartlett, M.D.

Professor of Medicine
Director, AIDS Service
Johns Hopkins University School of Medicine
Baltimore, Maryland

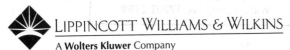

LIPPINCOTT WILLIAMS & WILKINS

A **Wolters Kluwer** Company

Philadelphia • Baltimore • New York • London
Buenos Aires • Hong Kong • Sydney • Tokyo

Managing Editor: Jennifer Jett
Compositor: Maryland Composition
Printer: Victor Graphics, Inc.

© **2005 by LIPPINCOTT WILLIAMS & WILKINS**
530 Walnut Street
Philadelphia, PA 19106 USA
LWW.com

Printed in the USA

ISBN: 0-7817-8911-7

First Edition, 1991	Fifth Edition, 1995	Ninth Edition, 2000
Second Edition, 1992	Sixth Edition, 1996	Tenth Edition, 2001
Third Edition, 1993	Seventh Edition, 1997	Eleventh Edition, 2003
Fourth Edition, 1994	Eighth Edition, 1998	Twelfth Edition, 2004

Care has been taken to confirm the accuracy of the information presented and to describe generally accepted practices. However, the authors, editors, and publisher are not responsible for errors or omissions or for any consequences from application of the information in this book and make no warranty, expressed or implied, with respect to the currency, completeness, or accuracy of the contents of the publication. Application of this information in a particular situation remains the professional responsibility of the practitioner.

The authors, editors, and publisher have exerted every effort to ensure that drug selection and dosage set forth in this text are in accordance with current recommendations and practice at the time of publication. However, in view of ongoing research, changes in government regulations, and the constant flow of information relating to drug therapy and drug reactions, the reader is urged to check the package insert for each drug for any change in indications and dosage and for added warnings and precautions. This is particularly important when the recommended agent is a new or infrequently employed drug.

Some drugs and medical devices presented in this publication have Food and Drug Administration (FDA) clearance for limited use in restricted research settings. It is the responsibility of the health care provider to ascertain the FDA status of each drug or device planned for use in their clinical practice.

01 02
1 2 3 4 5 6 7 8 9 10

PREFACE

The purpose of this publication is to provide guidelines for the care of patients with HIV infection. These recommendations reflect the policies of the AIDS Care Program at Johns Hopkins Hospital, where approximately 3000 patients with this infection are being followed. Recommendations for HIV care change frequently, so the care provider is cautioned that this guideline is dated July 2004. The twelfth edition has been augmented by additional tables and extensive revision of the text reflecting dramatic changes in treatment of HIV owing to advances in the field and the incredible complexity of care that accompanies these advances. This edition includes guidelines for management of HIV/AIDS from the Department of Health and Human Services for 2004.

For updated information visit our website: www.hopkins-aids.edu

CONTENTS

LIST OF TABLES AND FIGURES

TABLES

1—HIV Serology

Indications

Rapidly evolving improvements in medical care provide the incentive for increased serologic testing. The Centers for Disease Control (CDC) suggests that persons who are sexually active should be offered HIV serology.

Informed Consent

Testing should be voluntary with appropriate counseling. Informed consent is generally required, and some laboratories have policies that require the signature of the patient or the legal representative as a contingency for processing. An exception is that many states permit testing of the source with exposures to health care workers. Some areas offer anonymous testing in which all patient identifiers are removed. The usual charge for the test is $30–60; most state and local health departments offer HIV serology at no charge. There are 31 states that have required reporting of all persons with positive HIV serology. All states have mandatory reporting of AIDS cases.

Accuracy

Test results are reported as positive, negative, or indeterminate. The standard serologic test requires a positive enzyme-linked immunoabsorbent assay (ELISA) as a screening test and a positive Western blot (WB) for confirmation. The usual WB criteria are p24 plus glycoprotein (gp) 120/160 or gp 41 plus gp 120/160. Variations in diagnostic criteria and weak bands sometimes cause inconsistencies in reports, but this is unusual. The rate of <u>false-positive tests</u> is 0.0004–0.0007% (Arch Intern Med 2003;163:1857). The usual causes are technician error and HIV vaccines (Ann Intern Med 1994;121:584; JAMA 1998;280: 584). Factitious HIV infections refers to patients who erroneously claim this infection (Ann Intern Med 1994;121:763).

The frequency of <u>false-negative results</u> in a high-prevalence population (intravenous drug users [IDUs] with a seroprevalence rate of 30%) is about 0.3% (JID 1993;168:327), and in a low-prevalence population (blood donors) it is about 0.001% (NEJM

1

1991;325:1, 593). The usual cause of false-negative tests is testing during the time between transmission and seroconversion, a period that usually averages 10–12 days using newer tests (CID 1997;25:101; Am J Med 2000;160:3286). Other causes of false-negative results are agammaglobulinemia or infection with strains that are antigenically distinctive (Lancet 1996;348:176) such as HIV-2 (JAMA 1992;267:2775; Ann Intern Med 1993;118: 211) or the subtype O or subtype N of HIV-1 (Lancet 1993;343: 1393; MMWR 1996;45:561; Lancet 1994;344:1333). Subtypes O and N are extremely rare.

HIV-2 infection was reported in 78 patients in the U.S. from 1987 through January 1998, most of whom acquired the disease in West Africa (MMWR 1995;44:603). Standard enzyme immunoassay (EIA) screening assays used in the United States may include antigens to both HIV-1 and HIV-2; screening EIA tests for HIV-1 are positive in 70–80% of patients with HIV-2 infection, although WBs are often indeterminate or negative (JAMA 1992;267:2775; Ann Intern Med 1993;118:211). Testing for HIV-2 is recommended for patients from countries where HIV-2 is prevalent and those who are needle-sharing or sexual partners of such patients, persons who received transfusions in the endemic area, or children born of infected women. These countries include Benin, Burkina Faso, Ghana, Guinea, Nigeria, Liberia, Sao Tome, Senegal, Togo, Cape Verde, Ivory Coast, Gambia, Guinea-Bissau, Mali, Mauritania, and Sierra Leone. Only one case of HIV infection involving subtype O has occurred in the United States through July 1996 (MMWR 1996;45:561). Type N strains could also cause false-negative results, but there have been no cases of this infection in the United States (JID 2000;181:470). There are rare patients with persistently false-negative serologic tests (AIDS 1995;9:95; MMWR 1996;45:181; CID 1997;25:98; CID 1997;25:101).

The most common cause of <u>indeterminate results</u> is a positive ELISA and a single band on a WB. This may reflect late-stage disease, usually with loss of core antibody (p24 band). It may also reflect seroconversion where anti-p24 is usually the first to appear; the test should be repeated in 3–4 mo. Persons in low-risk categories with indeterminate test results are virtually never infected with either HIV-1 or HIV-2; repeat testing is likely to show persistence of indeterminate results, and the cause of this pattern is usually unknown (NEJM 1990;322:217). In view of the unnecessary anxiety evoked by knowledge of possible HIV infection, low-risk patients with indeterminate tests should be reassured that HIV infection is very unlikely, but the follow-up test is necessary to provide 100% assurance. When a non–antibody-dependent assay is necessary to confirm or clarify serologic assays, some authorities recommend the qualitative plasma HIV DNA polymerase chain reaction (PCR). This shows sensitivity of 97–98% and specificity of 98% (Ann Intern Med 1996;124:803), but the methods are now well-standardized and the reagents are not approved for this test.

Alternative Diagnostic Methods to Detect HIV

Alternative tests have been developed to increase access to testing (home test), to improve acceptability of testing (urine or salivary assays), and to reduce the time delay in availability of results (rapid tests), and to detect early infection (PCR test).

PCR Test.   This test is not advocated for screening due to a 2–9% rate of false-positives (Ann Intern Med 1999;130:37; J Clin Microbiol 2000;38:2837; Ann Intern Med 2001;134:25). These false-positives usually show low-level viral loads (<10,000 c/mL), so that high levels, as expected with acute HIV, became more valid indicators of infection. Thus, this becomes the preferred diagnostic test for acute HIV when sampling preceeds antibody response. This may also be used for screening by pairing PCR with standard serology to identify the subset with acute HIV; the goal is to intervene with disease prevention by contact tracing at the time the source is most likely to transmit HIV.

Home Tests.   The only Food and Drug Administration (FDA)-approved home test is the Home Access Express Test (Home Access Health Corporation, Hoffman Estates, IL; 800-HIV-TEST). The Home Access Test is available in pharmacies at $50–60/test. Blood is obtained by lancet; one drop is placed on a filter strip, and this is mailed using an anonymous code for patient identity. Testing consists of a double EIA screening test and a confirming immunoflourescence assay (IFA) test. Consumer telephones are provided for counseling, and the customer is instructed to call for results, which are available in ≤1 wk. Initial studies comparing home tests with standard serology show 100% sensitivity and 100% specificity (Arch Intern Med 1997;157:309). The advantage of this method is access to testing by some persons who are reluctant to use standard health care facilities. The main disadvantages are expense and concern for psychological reactions to results in a non-medical care environment.

Salivary test. OraSure (Epitope Co., Beaverton, OR; 888-ORA-SURE). A cotton pad is used to obtain saliva, which is placed in a vial and submitted to a laboratory for EIA and WB testing. A study of 3570 persons showed correct results compared with standard serology in 672 of 673 (99.9%) seropositives and 2893 of 2897 (99%) seronegatives (JAMA 1997;277:254). Results are available in 3 days by phone or fax. The cost is $24/test.

Urine test. Calypte HIV-1 Urine EIA (Calypte Inc., 510-749-5153). This test uses urine for EIA screening or dot blot assay (Genie HIV-1/HIV-2, Genetic Systems) (Eur J Clin Microbiol Infect Dis 1996;15:810). Positive results require confirmation by standard serology. The test is supplied as a 192-test kit for $816 or a 480-test kit for $1920; this translates to $4/test.

Rapid Tests.   There are three FDA-approved rapid tests: OraQuick Rapid HIV-1 Test, Reveal Rapid Antibody Test, and Uni-Gold Recombigen HIV test (www.cdc.gov/hiv/rapid_testing). Results are available in 20–30 minutes and show sensitivity and specificity rates >99% (J Clin Micro 2003;41:3868; J Lab Med 2003;27:288; Ann Intern Med 1999;131:4810). For all three tests, a negative result is considered a definitive negative unless tested in the "window period." Tests with positive results should be confirmed with Western blot or IFA. In terms of relative merit, the OraQuick test is "CLIA waved," which means there are no federal restrictions on personnel, quality control, or proficiency. The implication is that it can be "provider-read" at the site of testing, thus facilitating use in clinics, emergency rooms, etc. Rapid tests are particularly useful in settings where rapid results are a priority (occupational or non-occupational exposure, untested woman in labor) or a patient who is unlikely to return for routine serologic test results (as with STD clinics, Emergency rooms etc.).

2—Epidemiology (Table 1)

Current estimates are that the seroprevalence of HIV in the United States is 0.3%, and 900,000 persons are living with HIV infection (JAMA 1996;276:126); about 335,000 are receiving HIV care (NEJM 2001;344:817). The total reported with AIDS (1993 definition) for 1981 through December 2002 was 886,575 with 487,725 deaths (CDC Surveillance Supp Report vol 10, No. 1, 2004). The estimated number living with HIV/AIDS in 2002 was 384,906. Of these, 171,592 (45%) were gay men, 98,792 (26%) were injection drug users, 23,495 (6%) had both risks, and 80,147 (21%) reported heterosexual sex as the mechanism of transmission. Risk categories for 42,136 newly reported AIDS cases for 2002 follow: Gay men—42%, injection drug users—24%, both of these risks—5%, heterosexual contact—29%, and perinatal transmission—0.2% (90 cases).

Table 1. Seroprevalence of HIV in the United States

Category	Reference	Rate	Comment
Gay men	Am J Epidemiol 1987;126:568 J AIDS 1989;2:77 Science 1991;253:37 JAMA 1994;272:149 J AIDS 1995;9:514 AIDS Surveillance Report 13: No. 2;2002 Table 5 MMWR 2002;51:736 CDC AIDS Surveillance Report 10: No. 1, 2004	14–50%	• Average in Multicenter AIDS Cohort Study (5000 participants) was 36% at entry with 0.5–1.0% annual seroconversion rate; higher seroconversion rates are reported in young gay men • Gay men accounted for 16,944 of 42,136 (40%) of newly reported cases of AIDS reported in adults and adolescents in 2002 and 420,790 of 886,575 (47%) of cumulative cases reported through Dec 31, 2002 • The number of gay men with newly reported AIDS has been 16,076 to 17,357/year from 1998–2002
Intravenous drug users (IDUs)	JAMA 1989;261:2677 J AIDS 1993;6:1049 AIDS 1994;8:263 Arch Intern Med 1995;155:1305 CDC AIDS Surveillance Report 10: No. 1, 2004	1–60%	• Review of 92 studies showed great variation by location: New York City 34–61%; New Jersey 17–29%; Boston 28%; Puerto Rico 45–59%; Detroit 8–12%; San Francisco 5–16%; Miami 5%; New Orleans 1%; Atlanta 10%; Denver 1–5%; Los Angeles 2–5%; Minnesota 1%. Annual seroconversion rate: Baltimore 4%; LA nil; Philadelphia 2.5% in clients of methadone clinics and 14% in active users not in treatment • IDU accounted for 10,125 of 42,136 (24%) of newly reported cases of AIDS in adults and adolescents in 2002 and 240,268 of 886,575 (27%) of cumulative cases reported through December 31, 2002
Methadone clinic clients	NEJM 1992;326:375	1–30%	• Eight city surveys with rates ranging from 0.7% (Seattle) to 28.6% (Newark); average is 9%
Hemophilia (adults)	JAMA 1985;253:3409 J AIDS 1994;7:279 AIDS Surveillance Report 13: No. 2, 2002: Table 5 Ann Intern Med 2002;36:312	Type A 70% Type B 35%	• Applies primarily to hemophiliacs who received clotting factors before 1985. Hemophilia and 106 of 42,983 (0.2%) of newly reported AIDS cases in 2001 and a cumulative total of 5,292 of 807,075 (0.6%) cases reported through Dec 31, 2002

Group	References	Rate	Comments
Regular sex partners of HIV-infected persons	Arch Intern Med 1989;149:645 Am J Med 1988;85:472 JAMA 1991;266:1664 J AIDS 1993;6:497 Science 1995;270:1374 Am J Epidemiol 1997;146:350 NEJM 2000;342:921 Lancet 2001;357:1149 CDC AIDS Surveillance Report 10: No. 1, 2004	0–58%	• Average is 20–25% for wives of hemophiliac men with HIV infection • Discordant couple study in the U.S. showed efficiency of transmission 8:1 greater for male → female, but this was not seen in the discordant couple study in Africa where the ratio was 1:1 and the rate without protected sex was 0.001/ coital act. Rate of transmission is highly dependent on viral load, ranging from 0.0001/ coital act with VL < 1700 c/ml to 0.0023/coital act with VL > 38,500 c/ml. • Heterosexual transmission accounted for 12,413 of 42,136 (29%) of newly reported adult cases in 2002
Women (aged 18–59 yr)	Science 1995;270:1374 JAMA 1997;278:911 AIDS Surveillance Report 2002; 13:No. 2, Table 5	0.15%	• Women accounted for 10,955 of 42,136 (26%), newly reported AIDS cases in 2002. This compares with 534 of 8153 (7%) in 1985. Risk factors in reporting: IDU 3,180 (29%), heterosexual contact 7476 (68%)
Commercial sex workers	MMWR 1987;36:157 JAMA 1990;263:60	0–57%	• Great variation by location and confounding variable of IDU; Newark 57%; Washington DC 50%; Miami 19%; San Francisco 6%; Los Angeles 4%; Atlanta 1%; Las Vegas 0
College students Childbearing women and perinatal transmission	NEJM 1990;323:1538 JAMA 1991;265:1704 JAMA 1995;274:952	0.2% 0.15%	• Highest rates of HIV in pregnant woman were NYC 0.58%; Washington DC 0.55%; New Jersey 0.49%; Florida 0.45%
Pediatrics	NEJM 2002;346:1879 CDC AIDS Surveillance Report 10: No. 1, 2004		• Perinatal transmission rate without therapy is 25–30%, with azidothymidine (AZT) monotherapy is 8% and with highly active antiretroviral therapy (HAART) is 1–2% • Perinatal transmission accounted for 90 of 42,136 (0.2%) newly reported AIDS cases in 2002 and a cumulative total of 8,629 of 886,575 (1%) of all AIDS cases reported through 2002 • The number of perinatally acquired AIDS cases peaked in 1992 (905 cases) and decreased 90% to 90 cases in 2002

Table 1. (continued)

Category	Reference	Rate	Comment
Sexually transmitted disease (STD) clinic clients	STD 1992;19:235 J AIDS 1995;9:514 NEJM 1992;326:375	0.5–11%	• Summary of 552,665 serologic tests in 80 STD clinics from 1988–1992 showed HIV seroprevalence was 33% in gay men, 3% in heterosexual men, 2% in heterosexual women, and 10% in heterosexual injection drug users
Applicants to military	MMWR 1988;37:67 J AIDS 1990;3:1168 J AIDS 1995;10:177 JAMA 1991;265:1709	0.13%	• Annual seroconversion rate is 0.02–0.03%/yr
Transfusion recipients	NEJM 1995;333:1721 NEJM 1996;334:1685 Ann Intern Med 2002;136:312	0.02%	• Estimated 18–27 HIV transmissions/yr with blood transfusions in the United States • Transfusions accounted for 218 of 43,158 (0.2%) of newly reported AIDS cases in 2001 • Risk is 1 per 450,000–2 million units of screened blood
General population	Science 1991;253:37 MMWR 1990;30(RR-16) Science 1995;270:1374 MMWR 2002;51:736 CDC AIDS Surveillance Report 10: No. 1; 2004	0.4%	• Annual seroconversion rate in the United States based on assumption of 40,000 new infections/year is 0.016% • AIDS rates in 2002 in the US were 27/100,000 for men and 9/100,000 for women
Developing countries	BMJ 2001;322:1226 NEJM 2004;351:117	0.1–7.5%	• Prevalence in adults 18–49 yrs varies: Sub-Saharan Africa—7.5%; Southeast Asia—0.6%; Latin America—0.6%; Western Europe—0.3%; North America—0.6%; Middle East—0.2%. For globe prevalence is 1.1% • Risk for HIV in world: Blood transfusion 3–5%, perinatal transmission 5–10%, sex 70–80%, injection drug use 5–10% • The estimated total cases of persons living with HIV in 2003 was 37,800,000, including 25,000,000 (66%) in Sub-Saharan Africa, 6,500,000 (17%) in South and Southeast Asia, and 1,000,000 (2.6%) in North America

3—Classification and Natural History

Classification

The current CDC classification system (Table 2) uses three ranges of CD4 cell counts (>500, 200–499, and <200/mm^3) and a matrix of nine mutually exclusive categories. Category B includes most conditions previously classified as AIDS-related complex.

Natural History

Virologic Events and Immune Defense. HIV infection involves the complex interplay of viral replication and immune defenses. Clinical expression in early-stage disease (acute retroviral syndrome) is similar to other acute viral infections; characteristic features in late-stage disease reflect immune destruction, largely because of loss of CD4 cells, which are critical factors for modulating host defenses.

The sequence of events is the following: HIV is transmitted across the mucocutaneous barrier with extension to regional lymph tissue (days) → massive viremia with maximum plasma HIV RNA levels 2–4 wk after transmission expressed as the acute HIV syndrome; this is accompanied by a high risk of HIV transmission to others (JID 2004;189:1785), widespread dissemination, and extensive involvement of lymph tissue (weeks) → immune response with partial control ascribed to cytotoxic T-cell response (primarily CD8 cells) that is regulated by HIV-specific CD4 cytokine response and then with seroconversion (weeks-months) → persistent HIV replication with relatively constant levels of HIV RNA viremia after the "set point" is established about 4 mo after HIV transmission (Clin Infect Dis 2004;38:1447; NEJM 1998;339:33). Once the set point is reached the CD4 cell count gradually decreases, and viral load only slightly increases (JID 1999;180:1018). The CD4 decline that averages 50/mm^3/yr over a mean of 8–10 yr → massive destruction of immune system with susceptibility to opportunistic pathogens and opportunistic tumors when the CD4 cell count reaches <200/mm^3 (NEJM 1993;328:329) (Fig. 1).

The HIV replication rate in chronically infected patients ranges from 18 to 460/mm^3 and averages 10^{10} virions/day. The

Table 2. AIDS Surveillance Case Definition for Adolescents and Adults: 1993 (MMWR 1992;41:1–9)

CD4 Cell Categories	Clinical Categories		
	A Asymptomatic, Persistent Generalized Lymphadenopathy (PGL), or Acute HIV Infection	B Symptomatic (Not A or C)[b]	C[a] AIDS Indicator Condition (1987)
1. >500/mm^3 (≥29%)	A1	B1	C1
2. 200–499/mm^3 (14–28%)	A2	B2	C2
3. <200/mm^3 (<14%)	A3	B3	C3

[a] All patients in categories A3, B3, C1–C3 are reported as AIDS based on prior AIDS indicator conditions (see below) and/or a CD4 cell count of <200/mm^3. AIDS indicator conditions include three new entries added to the 1987 case definition (MMWR 1987;36:15): Recurrent bacterial pneumonia, invasive cervical cancer, and pulmonary tuberculosis.
[b] Symptomatic conditions not included in category C that 1) are attributed to HIV infection or indicate a defect in cell-mediated immunity or 2) are conditions considered to have a clinical course or to require management that is complicated by HIV infection. Examples of B conditions include but are not limited to bacillary angiomatosis; thrush; vulvovaginal candidiasis that is persistent, frequent, or poorly responsive to therapy; cervical dysplasia (moderate or severe); cervical carcinoma in situ; constitutional symptoms such as fever (38.5° C) or diarrhea for >1 mo; oral hairy leukoplakia; herpes zoster involving two episodes of >1 dermatome; ITP; listeriosis; pelvic inflammatory disease (PID) (especially if complicated by a tubo-ovarian abscess); peripheral neuropathy.

Indicator Conditions in Case Definition of AIDS

Candidiasis of esophagus, trachea, bronchi, or lungs
Cervical cancer, invasive[c,d]
Coccidioidomycosis, extrapulmonary[c]
Cryptococcosis, extrapulmonary
Cryptosporidiosis with diarrhea for >1 mo
Cytomegalovirus of any organ other than liver, spleen, or lymph nodes
Herpes simplex with mucocutaneous ulcer for >1 mo or bronchitis, pneumonitis, esophagitis
Histoplasmosis, extrapulmonary[c]
HIV-associated dementia[a]: disabling cognitive and/or motor dysfunction interfering with occupation or activities of daily living
HIV-associated wasting[c]: involuntary weight loss of >10% of baseline plus chronic diarrhea (≥2 loose stools/day for ≥30 days) or chronic weakness and documented enigmatic fever for ≥30 days
Isosporosis with diarrhea for >1 mo[c]
Kaposi's sarcoma in patient younger than 60 (or older than 60[c])
Lymphoma of brain in patient younger than 60 (or older than 60[c])
Lymphoma, non-Hodgkin's of B cell or unknown immunologic phenotype and histology showing small, noncleaved lymphoma or immunoblastic sarcoma
Mycobacterium avium or *M. kansasii,* disseminated
Mycobacterium tuberculosis, disseminated[c]
Mycobacterium tuberculosis, pulmonary[c,d]
Pneumocystis carinii pneumonia (PCP)
Pneumonia, recurrent-bacterial[c,d]
Progressive multifocal leukoencephalopathy
Salmonella septicemia (nontyphoid), recurrent[c]
Toxoplasmosis of internal organ

[c] Requires positive HIV serology.
[d] Added in the revised case definition 1993.

major target of HIV is CD4 cells, and cell destruction represents the effect of viral clearance by cytotoxic T lymphocytes (CTL) or "killer cells" (Nature 1993;366:22). Current estimates are that the average healthy adult harbors 10^{12} CD4 cells; approximately 10–25% of the CD4 population is infected early during HIV infection, and HIV infection results in destruction of about 10^9 CD4 cells/day. The implication is that 30% of the total body HIV burden turns over daily, and 6–7% of the CD4 cells turn over daily. These data are averages; kinetics of HIV and CD4 cells in individual patients are highly variable.

The course of the infection without therapy averages about 10 yr from the time of initial infection to an AIDS-defining diagnosis. In some patients, the rate of CD4 cell loss is rampant with counts of $<200/mm^3$ within 2 yr ("rapid progressors"); at the other extreme are "chronic nonprogressors"—defined as patients with HIV infection for >8 yr and CD4 counts of $>500/mm^3$, with no antiviral treatment (Lancet 1993;340:863). Sequential analysis of two cohorts followed from the time of seroconversion show a mean duration to CD4 counts of $<500/mm^3$ of 48 mo (Ann Intern Med 1996;125:257). In the Multicenter AIDS Cohort Study (MACS) cohort, 20 of 1800 (0.9%) had no significant decline in CD4 counts despite HIV infection for 14 yr with no antiretroviral therapy. These variations in course are thought to be dependent on the cytotoxic T cell (CD8 cell) response, which is ultimately dependent on competency of CD4 cells that regulate CD8 cells with HIV-specific CD4 cell responses and cytokines (Science 1997;278:1447; J Virol 1994;68:4650; Clin Infect Dis 2004;38:1447). The problem is the rapid consumption of CD4 cells by rapidly replicating HIV. The CD4 slope or rate of decline consequently depends on viral load and in one study showed a decrease of 4%/yr for each log_{10} HIV RNA/mL (JID 2002;185:905). The implication of these observations is that control of HIV replication in early stage disease (acute HIV syndrome) by natural defenses or HAART may lead to "long term nonprogression." Other factors that may influence the rate of progression follow:

- Defective virus (Lancet 1992;340:863): Rare
- Genetic susceptibility with lack of the CCR5 receptor site (Nature Med 1996;2:966; Emerg Infect Dis 1997;3:261)

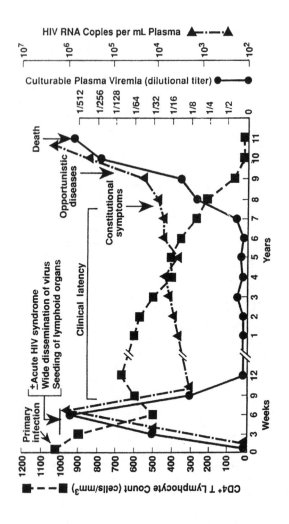

Figure 1. Typical course of HIV infection without therapy. The initial event is the acute retroviral syndrome accompanied by a decline in CD4 cell count (*squares*), high-level cultivable HIV plasma viremia (*circles*), and high plasma concentrations of HIV RNA (*triangles*) that reach zenith levels of 2–40 million copies/mL (JID 1999;180:1018). Clinical symptoms usually resolve spontaneously in 1–3 wk; this recovery is accompanied by a rapid decline in plasma viremia, reflecting CTL response (Science 1996;272:505; Science 1997;278:1447). The CD4 cell count may return toward baseline, although some studies show no rebound (Ann Intern Med 1996;125:257) and then show a linear decline that averages 50/mm^3/yr. The subsequent course generally shows a prolonged period of clinical latency that is accompanied by high rates of HIV replication with an average of approximately 10^{10} new virions/day. Plasma concentrations of HIV RNA predict the course (about 10^3/mL for slow progressors and >10^5/mL for rapid progressors) (Ann Intern Med 1997;126:946). The CD4 cell count decline (CD4 slope) is often accelerated during late-stage disease as indicated by the ``inflection point'' of the CD4 slope, and this is accompanied by increased levels of HIV RNA. A CD4 cell count of 200/mm^3 is generally regarded as the threshold at which patients become vulnerable to opportunistic infections. The median time to an AIDS-defining complication after reaching 200/mm^3 is 18–24 mo; the median survival after a CD4 count of 200/mm^3 is 3.1 yr; and the median survival after an AIDS-defining complication is 1.3 yr. (This is without antiretroviral therapy.) With no therapy directed against HIV and no PCP prophylaxis, the average time from viral transmission to an AIDS-defining diagnosis is about 10 yr. Data provided for the CD4 cell count decline are averages based on natural history studies in the Multicenter AIDS Cohort Study (MACS) (JID 1993;168:149; J AIDS 1995;8:66). There is substantial individual variation; some patients have a rapid decline in CD4 cell counts after acute retroviral syndrome, and 5–15% are considered chronic nonprogressors with CD4 cell counts exceeding 500/mm^3 for more than 8 yr (J AIDS 1995;8:496). Given comparable care, there is no significant difference in rates of progression based on sex, race, or risk category. Variations in rates of progression in untreated adults correlate primarily with host defense, especially CTL response that is regulated by the HIV-specific CD4 cell response (Science 1996;271:324; PNAS 1997;94:254; Science 1997;278:1447; Lancet 2004;363:863). (Fig. 1 is reproduced with permission from Ann Intern Med 1996;124:654; JID 1999;180:1018.)

- Age: Duration of survival is inversely correlated with age (Lancet 1996;347:1573; Lancet 2000;355:1131). Note that other demographic characteristics (gender, race, risk, etc.) do not seem to influence rates of progression
- Major histocompatibility genes (Nature Med 1996;4:405; Hosp Pract 1998;33:53)
- Plasma level of HIV RNA after the set point is established (Science 1996;272:1167; Ann Intern Med 1997;126:946; JID 2000;181:872)
- Cytotoxic T-lymphocyte (CTL) response appears to be the critical determinant of viral load set point and rate of progression (Science 1997;278:1447; Clin Infect Dis 2004;38:1447)

Medical interventions that are associated with a significant increase in survival:

1. Antiretroviral therapy (NEJM 1998;338:853; Lancet 1998; 252:1725; Lancet 2003;362:1267; Lancet 2003;362:877)
2. *P. carinii* prophylaxis (JAMA 1988;259:118)
3. *M. avium* prophylaxis (NEJM 1996;335:384)
4. Care by a physician with HIV experience (NEJM 1996;334:701; JAIDS 2000;24:106; J Gen Intern Med 2003;18:95; Ann Intern Med 1999;13:136)

Viral transmission. The efficiency of HIV transmission with discordant couples without antiviral therapy or condoms is estimated to be about 0.2% (Lancet 2001;357:1149). This estimate is based on a longitudinal survey of discordant couples in Uganda; the actual frequency of transmission was 1/558 acts of sexual intercourse (NEJM 2000;342:921). The risk with a needlestick injury from an HIV-infected source is about 0.3% or about 1/300 (Ann Intern Med 1990;113:740). The rate for perinatal transmission is about 23% with vaginal delivery (NEJM 1996;335:1621). All of these rates are highly correlated with the viral load in the source (NEJM 1999;341:394; Lancet 2001;357:1149; AIDS 2001;15:621; JID 2001;183:206). Analysis of the study of discordant couples indicated the risk of transmission increased about 2.5-fold for each log 10 c/mL increase in viral load (NEJM 2000;340:921). These findings emphasize the relative efficiency of HIV transmission with the acute HIV syndrome when viral loads are especially high, a risk that is "brief but efficient" (JID 2004;189:1785).

Table 3. Acute HIV Infection

Symptomatic disease: 50–89%
Frequency of correct diagnosis with medical consultation: 25%
Incubation period (HIV exposure to onset of symptoms): 2–6 wk
Symptoms and signs

Fever	96%	Diarrhea	32%
Adenopathy	74%	Nausea or vomiting	27%
Pharyngitis	70%	Hepatosplenomegaly	14%
Rash[a]	70%	Thrush	12%
Myalgias	54%	Neurologic symptoms[b]	12%
Headache	32%		

Duration of symptoms (mean): 1–3 wk
Laboratory tests: Plasma viremia with high titer (peak of 2–40 million copies/
  mL). HIV-1 serologic test negative or indeterminant

Adapted from JID 1993;168:1490; Ann Intern Med 1996;125:257; CID 1998;26:323; JID 1997;
176:112; JAIDS 2002;31:318.
[a] Erythematous maculopapular rash involving the face, trunk, and extremities ± soles
and palms. There may be mucocutaneous ulcerations involving the mouth, esophagus,
or genitals.
[b] Includes aseptic meningitis, meningoencephalitis, peripheral neuropathy, facial
palsy. Guillain-Barré syndrome, brachial neuritis, cognitive impairment, or psychosis.

Acute HIV infection.   It is estimated that 40–90% of acutely
infected patients will have an associated clinical illness (Clin
Infect Dis 2004;38:1447; Ann Intern Med 1997;126:174). This illness generally occurs 1–3 wk after an exposure such as a
needlestick injury in a health care worker or sexual exposure
(Ann Intern Med 1996;125:257; Ann Intern Med 1993;118:913;
JID 1994;168:1490). The time to seroconversion after viral transmission, which is usually within 3–12 wk, has been reported as
long as 6–12 months (Am J Med 1997;102:117; NEJM 1998;339:
33).

Clinical features (Table 3) are those of an infectious mononu-
cleosis-like illness with fever, adenopathy, hepatosplenomeg-
aly, sore throat, myalgias, morbilliform rash, mucocutaneous
ulceration, diarrhea, and leukopenia with atypical lymphocytes
(Ann Intern Med 1993;118:913; JID 1994;168:1490; Ann Intern
Med 1996;125:257; CID 1998; 26:323). Some patients have neurologic symptoms such as aseptic meningitis, Guillain-Barré syndrome, or acute psychosis. The five most common clinical features in the Seattle study were fever (mean 38.9°C), sore throat,
fatigue, malaise, and weight loss (average 5 kg); 17% were hospi-
talized and 24% had signs of aseptic meningitis (Ann Intern

Med 1996;125:257). Important clues that help distinguish this condition from other similar viral infections are the rash, mucosal ulcerations, generalized adenopathy neurologic abnormalities, and weight loss. The febrile illness is self-limited, usually lasting 1–3 wk.

Laboratory studies may show leukopenia and increased transaminase levels. Serologic tests for HIV are negative. The diagnosis is best established by HIV viral load (which is 100% sensitive and 90% specific) (Ann Intern Med 2001;134:25). The usual test in primary HIV is plasma HIV RNA. There are false-positives with this assay but only at low titer; the usual titer expected is >10,000 copies/mL. This is an important issue because this early period may be associated with a particularly high rate of transmission and because aggressive treatment of primary HIV infection may be the optimal time to influence the disease course (JID 2001;183:1466).

Seroconversion. Seroconversion generally takes place 3–12 wk after transmission (JAMA 1998;280:1080; Am J Med 2000;109:568; Clin Infect Dis 2004;38:1447). The CTL response precedes humoral response and is accompanied by a sharp reduction in plasma concentrations of HIV RNA copies (PNAS 1997;94:254) and resolution of symptoms of acute HIV infection.

Establishment of HIV RNA plasma level set point. Plasma levels of HIV RNA are established at a set point that is relatively stable over several years characterized as "chronic asymptomatic HIV infection." During this time there is a gradual increase in mean HIV RNA levels averaging about 7%/yr (Ann Intern Med 1998;128:613) with occassional blips reflecting antigenic stimuli (intercurrent illness or immunizations) (Ann Intern Med 1996;125:257; Ann Intern Med 1997;126:946). This set point dictates the subsequent rate of progression: High concentrations (>100,000 copies/mL) are associated with a CD4 slope of -76 cells/mm^3/yr and a median survival of 4.4; low concentrations (<5000 copies/mL) are associated with a CD4 slope of -36 cells/mm^3/yr and a median survival exceeding 10 yr (Ann Intern Med 1997;126:946).

Symptomatic HIV infection. Complications of HIV infection are ascribed to direct effects of the virus and to the consequences of immunosuppression:

- Direct effect of HIV: Acute HIV syndrome, persistent generalized lymphadenopathy (PGL), HIV-associated dementia, lymphocytic interstitial pneumonia (LIP), HIV-associated nephropathy, and progressive immunosuppression. Other possible consequences are anemia, neutropenia, thrombocytopenia, cardiomyopathy, myopathy, peripheral neuropathy, chronic meningitis, polymyositis, and Guillain-Barré syndrome.
- Immunosuppression results in opportunistic infections and tumors, primarily reflecting compromised cell-mediated immunity.

The correlation between these complications and the CD4 count as a barometer of immunocompetence is summarized in Table 5. In each instance the CD4 stratum assigned is the highest in which the designated complication is likely to be encountered; virtually all conditions increase in frequency with progressive decline in CD4 count.

Early complications generally represent complications of HIV infection per se, or they are infections involving relatively virulent microbes that do not require severe immunosuppression for clinical expression. The latter include vaginal candidiasis, pneumococal pneumonia, tuberculosis, and zoster. The complications designated as AIDS-defining (Table 5) generally occur with severe immunosuppression to CD4 counts below $200/mm^3$ and usually below $100/mm^3$. The relative frequency of these complications as the original AIDS-defining diagnosis is summarized in Table 4, and their frequency as a cause of death in the pre-HAART era is summarized in Table 6.

Asymptomatic infection. During this period the patient is asymptomatic or may have persistent generalized lymphadenopathy. There is usually a gradual decline in the CD4 cell count in untreated patients averaging 40–$60/mm^3/yr$, but with substantial individual differences based on viral load and variations in the test in the test (JID 1992;165:352). The first AIDS-defining opportunistic infection occurs with an average CD4 count of $70/mm^3$ (Am J Epidemiol 1995;141:645). Note that these data on natural history are based on studies of patients who had no antiretroviral therapy. The experience with the history of HIV in patients receiving HAART is dramatically different.

Table 4. Correlation of Complications with CD4 Cell Strata

CD4 Cell Count[a]	Infections[b]	Noninfectious Complications
>500/mm³	Acute HIV syndrome *Candida* vaginitis	Persistent generalized lymphadenopathy (PGL) Polymyositis Aseptic meningitis Guillain-Barré syndrome
200–500/mm³	Pneumococcal and other bacterial pneumonia (90) Pulmonary TB (90–180) Kaposi sarcoma (30–130) Herpes zoster (150–170) Thrush Cryptosporidiosis, self-limited Oral hairy leukoplakia	Cervical intraepithelial neoplasia Cervical cancer (180) Lymphocytic interstitial pneumonitis (100–500) Mononeuronal multiplex Anemia Idiopathic thrombocytopenic purpura
<200/mm³	*P. carinii* pneumonia (40–120) *Candida* esophagitis (30–80) Disseminated/chronic herpes simplex (40–110) Toxoplasmosis (20–40) Cryptococcosis (20–60) Disseminated histoplasmosis (30) Disseminated coccidioidomycosis (40) Cryptosporidiosis, chronic (40–130) Progressive multifocal leukoencephalopathy (PML) (40–110) Microsporidiosis (20–100) Miliary/extrapulmonary TB (40)	Wasting (20–100) B-cell lymphoma (30–60) Cardiomyopathy (25) Peripheral neuropathy (30–100) HIV-associated dementia (20–60) CNS lymphoma (20) HIV-associated nephropathy (20)
<50/mm³	CMV disease (10–20) Disseminated *M. avium* complex (10–20)	

[a] Indicated complications occur with increased frequency at lower CD4 strata; lymphomas may occur at any CD4 cell strata but are most frequent with counts <200/mm.³
[b] Number in parentheses indicates approximate median CD4 cell count at the time of diagnosis (see CID 1995;21 (Suppl 1):56; JAMA 1992;267:1798; Ann Intern Med 1996;124:633). Some values are ranges indicating multiple sources. (CDC, MACS (A. Munoz, personal communication).)

Table 5. Frequency of Initial AIDS-Defining Diagnosis

	Initial AIDS Defining Diagnosis[a]			Frequency Among All Patients (%)[b]
	1990 (%)	1995 (%)	1997 (%)	
Pneumocystis carinii pneumonia	49	28	42	75–85
HIV wasting syndrome	17	14	11	70–90
Candida esophagitis	13	11	15	20–30
Kaposi's sarcoma	11	6	11	15–25
HIV-associated dementia	6	4	4	40–70
Disseminated CMV	6	6	4	80–90
Toxoplasmosis encephalitis	5	3	3	5–15
Disseminated *M. avium* infection	4	4	5	30–40
Lymphoma	3	2	4	3–5
Chronic mucocutaneous herpes simplex	3	4	1	10–25
Cryptococcal meningitis	3	4	—	8–12
Cryptosporidiosis	2	2	2	5–10
Tuberculosis	—	5[c]	5	4–20

[a] Frequency according to CDC criteria for AIDS 1987–1992 as reported for newly diagnosed cases in 1990 and for 1995.
[b] Estimated lifetime frequency among all patients with AIDS without prophylaxis.
[c] Added in the revised case definition of 1993.

Table 6. Causes of Death in U.S. Patients Dying of AIDS

	1987 $n = 10,001$ (%)	1992 $n = 24,230$ (%)	1997–8* $n = 903$ (%)
Pneumonia—unspecified cause	18	18	—
P. carinii pneumonia	33	14	6
Non-tuberculosis (TB) mycobacteria	7	12	6
Bacterial septicemia	9	12	9
Kaposi's sarcoma	12	10	9
CMV disease	5	10	9
Non-Hodgkin's lymphoma	4	6	11
Toxoplasmosis	5	5	1
Cryptococcosis	8	5	3
TB	3	4	—
PML	1	2	2

* Data for San Francisco (JID 2002; 186:1019).

4—Patient Evaluation

Summary of Guidelines of U.S. Public Health Service—Infectious Diseases Society of America (MMWR 2002;51 RR-7); www.aidsinfo.nih.gov//guidelines)

Initial Evaluation

1. *Medical history.* Obtain a complete medical history with emphasis on the following.
   a. *HIV serology.* Dates of positive and negative tests; necessity to confirm a positive test; reason for prior HIV test
   b. *Transmission category.* Gay male, injection drug use, heterosexual contact, transfusion, hemophilia, other or unknown
   c. *HIV-related history.* CD4 cell counts, history of AIDS-defining diagnoses
   d. *Medical care.* Usual source and care, prior purified protein derivatives (PPDs), Papanicolaou (Pap) smear, vaccinations (HBV, influenza, Pneumovax, tetanus HAV)
   e. *Past medical history.* Cardiovascular disease and risks for cardiovascular disease (obesity, smoking, hypertension, diabetes, family history, blood lipids). Other: Pulmonary, renal, skin, hepatic, neurologic, urologic/gynecologic, gastrointestinal, surgeries, hospitalizations
   f. *Targeted conditions relevant to HIV.* TB exposure/risk; prior chickenpox or shingles; sexually transmitted diseases; hepatitis A, B, or C; gynecologic/obstetric history; alcoholism, drug use
   g. *Medications.* For HIV, for non-HIV medical conditions, over-the-counter drugs, alternative or complementary medicine; history of compliance with HIV medications and other medications
   h. *Review of systems.* Constitutional: Weight loss, fever, night sweats, fatigue; gastrointestinal (GI): Anorexia, dysphagia, nausea, vomiting, diarrhea, abdominal pain; chest: chest pain, dyspnea, cough; neurological: headaches,

weakness, painful extremeties, mental status changes, paresthesias; miscellaneous: Rashes, insomnia, adenopathy, vision

2. *Patient education.* Determine HIV risk behavior and assess ongoing high-risk behavior that places patient contacts at risk. Are patients placed at risk aware of this risk? Patient education should include discussion of safe sex, safe use of needles for injection drug users, risk of childbearing, and need to test patients placed at risk. Notification of contacts is often performed by the local health department without identification of the source, or notification may be an option offered the patient; regulations are variable in different states. All patients should be aware of the advances in HIV therapy that took place in 1996 because they revolutionized HIV care and dramatically changed outcome; they should also know that cure is unlikely with the currently available drugs.

3. *Patient examination* including the following:

   Oropharynx
   Lymphadenopathy
   Skin
   Heart and lungs
   Abdomen
   Genital/pelvic
   Neurologic

4. *Laboratory tests*
   - *HIV serology* (confirm prior test if necessary—should have documentation of positive serology, AIDS-defining diagnosis, or positive HIV RNA level)
   - *CBC*
   - *CD4 count*
   - *Quantitative plasma HIV RNA*
   - *Chemistry profile* including renal function and liver function tests
   - *Toxoplasma serology (IgG)*
   - *Chest x-ray* (utility of a baseline chest x-ray is questionable in patients with a negative PPD (Arch Intern Med 1996;156:191))
   - *PPD* (unless history of positive PPD or history of TB treatment; *Mycobacterium bovis* (BCG) does not preclude meaningful test results)

- *STD screen;* rapid plasma reagin (RPR) or Venereal Disease Research Laboratory Test (VDRLT), gonococcus (GC) and chlamydia urine screen using nucleic acid amplification tests (NAATs); this is advocated for sexually active patients (MMWR 2002;51 (RR-15):1)
- *Baseline fasting lipid profile and glucose* in all candidates for HAART therapy
- *Hepatitis screen:* Anti-HBc (to determine candidates for HBV vaccine or anti-HBs if previously vaccinated); HBsAg and anti-HCV (to detect active hepatitis if unexplained elevated transaminase levels; anti-HCV in all injection drug users)
- *Pap smear* (if none in past year)
- Optional tests: CMV serology (sometimes advocated for patients in low CMV risk categories), HAV antibody (advocated as a means to avoid unnecessary HAV vaccine in HCV co-infected patients who are candidates for HAV vaccine), varicella antibody (if no history of chickenpox), G6PD (sometimes done at baseline in patients with high risk: African Americans and men of Mediterranean heritage)

5. *Sequential tests*

   HIV RNA plasma levels: Baseline, confirmatory test at 2–4 wk, then every 3 mo if stable or more frequently with initiation of antiretroviral therapy or change in therapy or to confirm/refutte outlier

   CD4 count: Baseline and then every 3–6 mo ± confirmatory test if outlier result

   PPD: Annual in high-risk patients with persistently negative results

   VDRL or RPR: Annual in sexually active patients

   Pap smear: Baseline 6 mo, and then annually if negative

   Complete blood count (CBC): Baseline and every 3–6 mo (as a component of CD4 count)

6. *Drug toxicity monitoring*

   AZT–CBC every 3 mo (or more frequently if anemia or neutropenia)

   ddC, ddI, d4T—peripheral neuropathy including history and ankle jerks

   Nevirapine–liver function tests baseline, 2 and 4 wk, then monthly × 3 mo, then every 3 mo.

Protease inhibitors ± NNRTI—fasting lipid profile (cholesterol, low-density lipoprotein [LDL], high-density lipoprotein [HDL], triglycerides) at baseline and in 3–6 mo; subsequent frequency depends on risks and test results. Fasting levels necessary for triglycerides are used to determine LDL; should be done after 8- to 12-hr fast.

7. *Consultations* (all are optional)

Psychiatry

Obstetrics and gynecology

Ophthalmology: Sometimes advocated for all patients with a CD4 count <100/mm^3 at 6-mo intervals

Nutrition

8. *Vaccines*

Pneumococcal vaccine: Recommended for patients with CD4 count >200/mm; consider in those with CD4 count <200, for those with vaccination ≥5 yr previously, and for those vaccinated with CD4 count <200 who had immune reconstitution

Influenza: Recommended; response reduced with CD4 <200/mm^3; revaccinate annually October–November

HBV vaccine: Generally recommended for those at risk with negative anti-HBVc or anti-HBVs

HAV vaccine: All patients at risk (negative anti-HAV) plus high-risk category (MSM, illegal drug users) and those with chronic liver disease

Tetanus booster: Should be given every 10 yr

Resources for Providers and Patients

Provider Information Resources. Resources for patient management information for providers include the following.

Guidelines of the U.S. Public Health Service and Department of Health and Human Services. http://aidsinfo.nih.gov

1. Antiretroviral Therapy for Adults and Adolescents: MMWR 2002;51[RR-7]; (Updated version on website 3/27/04)

2. Occupational Exposure: MMWR 2001;50(RR-11) and National Clinician's PEP Hotline (CDC) 888-448-4911 or http://www.ucsf.edu/hivcntr (Updated version expected in Aug/Sept 2004)

3. Prevention of Opportunistic Infections: MMWR 2002;51[RR-6]

4. Prevention of HIV Transmission (Clin Infect Dis 2004;38:104; MMWR 2002;51 RR-15)
5. Antiretroviral Agents in Pregnancy: MMWR 2002;51[RR-7]; (Updated version 6/23/04)

Other Sources

1. Antiretroviral Treatment for adult HIV infection in 2002 IAS-USA (JAMA 2004;292:251)
2. British HIV Association Guidelines for the Treatment of HIV Infected Adults with Antiretroviral Therapy (http://www.bhiv.org) (July 2003)
3. Antiretroviral Drug Resistance Testing in Adults Infected with HIV: 2003 Recommendations of IAS-USA (Clin Infect Dis 2003;37:113) (Updated-Top HIV Med 11:215 Nov–Dec 2003)
4. Guidelines for Evaluation and Management of Dyslipidemia in HIV-infected Adults Receiving Antiretroviral Therapy: Recommendations of IDSA and AACTG (Clin Infect Dis 2003; 37:613)

AIDS Education Training Centers

An HRSA sponsored consortium of 17 regional HIV/AIDS education centers in the United States to target HIV providers with emphasis on medical management; activities include a National Minority Center to facilitate access by disenfranchised patients and a National Resource Center to promote DHHS guidelines.

Websites for AIDS/HIV Medical Information

www.hopkins-aids.edu (Johns Hopkins University)
www.medscape.com (MedScape)
www.healtheon.com
http://hivinsite.ucsf.edu (University of California at San Francisco)
www.healthdatabase.com/AIDS.htm (general information resource through linkages)
www.cdcnpin.org (CDC news)
www.sfaf.org/treatment (New developments and treatment)
www.aegis.org (Daily HIV briefing)
www.hivandhepatitis.com (HIV-Hepatitis co-infection)

Patient Information Resources.   Multiple information resources are available to patients that vary in content, quality, timeliness, sophistication (reading level), and language (English and Spanish primarily). The most reliable sources follow.

PWP Coalition of New York.   50 West 17th Street, New York, NY; publishes monthly "PWP Coalition Newsletter" about alternative medicines and outreach activities: 212-647-1415

Local AIDS services.   A national directory with a listing of services by geographic location from the U.S. Conference of Mayors, 1620 Eye Street, NW, Washington, DC 20006 ($15): 202-293-7330

Patient forum.   More than 2000 questions and answers in lay language available from Dr. Joel Gallant on the Johns Hopkins HIV website, which is also the recommended website for general patient education on HIV: www.hopkins-aids.edu

HIV/AIDS treatment information service.   A Public Health Service free telephone reference service for patients and providers; offers extensive library of patient information: 800-448-0440 or write PO Box 6303, Rockville, MD 20849-6303; www.hivatis.org

Therapeutic trials hotline.   National Institute of Allergy and Infectious Diseases: 1-800-TRIALS-A

American Foundation for AIDS Research (AmFar).   "AIDS/HIV Experimental Treatment Directory" (updated quarterly) and "AIDS Targeted Information Newsletter": 212-682-7440 ($125/year), www.amfar.org

Gay Men's Health Crisis (GMHC).   "Treatment Issues," GMHC, Department of Medical Information, 129 West 20th Street, New York, NY 10011: 212-807-6655 ($30/year; reliable reviews of therapeutics); Department of Education and Advocacy, 212-337-3505

National AIDS hotline.   Contracted through CDC for general information including local services: English (24 hr/day, 7 days/wk) 800-342-AIDS; Spanish (8:00 AM–2:00 PM, 7 days/wk) 1-800-344-SIDA; deaf (10:00 AM–10:00 PM, Mon–Fri) 1-800-243-7889

CDC National Prevention Information Network (HIV, STDs, TB).   A library for information with publications, videos, lists of services, and community-based organizations, PO Box 6303, Rockville, MD 20849-6303: 800-458-5231

Guide to Living with HIV Infection.   2001 (4th ed), Johns Hopkins University Press, 2715 North Charles Street, Baltimore, MD 21218-4319 (paperback $15.95)

University of California at San Francisco AIDS Health Project.   Psychotherapy, substance abuse counseling, HIV testing, support groups, 1855 Folsom St, Suite 670, San Francisco, CA 94103, 415-476-3902, www.ucsf-ahp.org

Bulletin of Experimental Treatments for AIDS (BETA).   San Francisco AIDS Foundation; request from BETA Subscriber Services, Infocom Group, 1250 45th Street, Suite 200, Emoryville, CA 94608-2924: 800-959-1059 ($75/year; trial subscription without payment offered [suggested for the sophisticated reader])

Legal issues/civil rights.   Office of Civil Rights, Department of Health and Human Services, PO Box 13716, Mail Stop 07, Philadelphia, PA 19101: 215-596-6109; social security—disability qualifications: 800-772-1213

National Institute on Drug Abuse hotline.   Substance abuse referral and printed material resource: English 800-662-4357; Spanish 800-662-9832

Project Inform.   HIV treatment information, treatment hotline and advocacy with publications and services. 1-800-822-7422, www.projinf.org

National Association of People with AIDS.   NAPWA 1413 K St NW, 7th floor Wash DC 20005 www.napwa.org 202-898-0414. Information about local resources, including support groups, mail order pharmacy, update information on new treatments, and two quarterly publications: "Medical Alert" (treatments) and "Active Voice" (advocacy)

"Wellness": Exercise, Smoking, Alcohol.   Medical care should include appropriate attention to nutrition, exercise, continued work, and other facets of "wellness." Depression does not appear to accelerate disease progression (JAMA 1993;270: 2563). Three separate studies have demonstrated deleterious consequences of smoking with increased rates of PCP and more rapid progression to AIDS (AIDS 1990;4:327; NEJM 2003;349: 1993; Chest 2003;123:1977). It is unknown whether effective *Pneumocystis carinii pneumoniae* (PCP) prophylaxis would nullify the disadvantage. Strenuous exercise as done by Olympic athletes or marathon runners is deleterious to immune function with increased susceptibility to common viral infections but is not known to reduce cell-mediated immunity; moderate exercise such as jogging or bicycle riding has no apparent adverse effect on immune function and may improve sense of well-being. Alcohol in moderation (one drink per day) has no adverse health consequences including problems with immune function, infections, rates of liver disease, or rates of hepatotoxicity with isoniazid, PIs, etc.; obviously, alcohol may reduce inhibitions and enhance high-risk behavior and also promote side effects of psychiatric or sedative drugs. Of particular concern is the effect alcohol has on compliance with complex medical regimens, especially binge drinking. HIV and alcohol are the two-way cofactors adding risk of progression with HCV; HIV-infected patients with HCV or HBV co-infection should not drink alcohol at all. Nutrition needs emphasis, but it is unknown whether routine nutrition consults, specific diets, vitamin supplements, or mineral supplements are advantageous (Lancet 1991;338:86; Nutr Rev 1990;48:393). Unusual diets such as macrobiotic diet and megavitamins may be dangerous. Multivitamin supplements have been found to delay HIV progression in a controlled trial in Tanzania (NEJM 2004;351:23).

Role of Pets, Food, Travel, and Occupational Risks
(Ann Intern Med 1997;127:939)

Pets.   The major concern with pets is that they may carry the microbes that cause diarrhea in patients, primarily *Cryptosporidia*, *Salmonella*, and *Campylobacter*. The following precautions help avoid this type of exposure and are relevant primarily to those with a CD4 count <200/mm^3: Veterinary consultation should be obtained if the pet develops diarrhea. When obtaining a new pet, avoid animals younger than 6 mo, pets with diarrhea, stray animals, and animals from facilities that have poor hygienic conditions. Wash hands after handling pets and especially before eating, and avoid contact with stool. If a pet develops diarrhea, it should be examined by a veterinarian.

Cats are of particular concern owing to risk of exposure to toxoplasmosis and *Bartonella*, as well as the microbes that cause diarrhea. It is best to obtain a cat older than 1 yr that is in good health. Litter boxes should be cleaned daily, preferably by someone who is not infected with HIV nor is pregnant. If this must be done by an HIV-infected person, hands should be washed thoroughly afterward to reduce the risk. Cats should be kept indoors, should not hunt, and should not be fed raw or undercooked meat because all of these increase the risk of toxoplasmosis. *Bartonella* is transmitted by bites and scratches of cats, and these should be avoided and should be cleaned promptly when they occur. It is not suggested to declaw a cat or test the animal for either toxoplasmosis or *Bartonella* infection.

With regard to other pets, healthy birds may be the source of cryptococcus or *Histoplasma*. Reptiles such as snakes and turtles may carry *Salmonella*. Aquariums are generally safe, but gloves should be used for cleaning to reduce exposure to *Mycobacterium marinum*. Nonhuman primates such as monkeys should be avoided.

Food.   The major risk with food and fluids is exposure to the microbes that cause diarrhea. Most enteric pathogens cause diarrhea in any host after exposure. The two that are particularly problematic to patients with AIDS are cryptosporidiosis, which can cause debilitating and chronic diarrhea in those with a CD4 count of $<180/mm^3$ and *Salmonella*, which commonly causes bacteremia in AIDS. *Salmonella* is often present in eggs and poultry, and undercooked meat is a common source of toxoplasmosis. The usual recommendation is to avoid raw or undercooked eggs, including the foods that often contain raw eggs such as hollandaise sauce and Caesar salad dressing. Also avoid raw or undercooked poultry, seafood, and meat. Poultry and meat should be cooked until they are no longer pink in the middle. Produce should be washed thoroughly before it is eaten. Patients should be reminded of the possibility of exposure to undercooked meats or other products through contact with cutting boards, counters, knives, and hands used in preparation; all should be washed carefully.

Warn patients to not drink directly from lakes or rivers because of the risk of cryptosporidiosis. There are sometimes community outbreaks of diarrhea in which there is a "boil-water" advisory. At such a time the water should be boiled 1 min to remove the risk of *Cryptosporidium* and other disease-causing microbes. Other options are submicron personal-use water filters and/or bottled water. The submicron filter recommended is one that is labeled "absolute" 1-μm filter; the best are those labeled to show they meet National Sanitation Foundation Standard number 53 for "cyst removal." Note that many filters labeled 1 μm are not standardized and are consequently not recommended. It is not generally recommended that HIV-infected persons boil the water or use tap water filtration if there is no advisory, but some may choose to use these precautions to be extra cautious.

Travel   (CID 2000;31:1403). The greatest health risk to persons with and without HIV infection is visits to developing countries, and the major problem is microbes that contaminate food and water. Avoid raw fruits and vegetables, raw or undercooked seafood or meat, tap water, ice made from tap water, nonpasteurized milk and dairy products, and items purchased from street vendors. The preferred foods are those that are steaming hot, fruits that can be peeled by the traveler, bottled water, hot coffee or tea, or anything with alcohol in it. Water may also be treated with iodine or chlorine, but this is not as effective as a rolling boil for 1 min. These recommendations apply to all travelers regardless of HIV status (CID 2000;32:331).

Antibiotics to prevent infections during travel to developing countries are usually not recommended, but they may be for some HIV-infected patients who are considered at high risk. A common recommendation is for a fluoroquinolone to prevent or treat diarrhea. Trimethoprim-sulfamethoxazole (TMP-SMX) is sometimes used, which many travelers may already be taking to prevent *Pneumocystis* pneumonia. It is important to be aware of the side effects of TMP-SMX when taken for prophylaxis during travel because these may appear to be some tropical disease. The most common reaction is a rash and fever, and the only treatment necessary is to simply stop the drug. For travelers to developing countries who do not take antibiotics, it is generally recommended to take loperamide for the treatment of mild diarrhea (≤ 2 loose stools/24 hr) or loperamide plus a fluoroquinolone for more severe diarrhea or diarrhea associated with fever and constitutional symptoms. The standard dose of loperamide is 4 mg, then 2 mg with each loose stool for a maximum of 16 mg/day. The dose of ciprofloxacin is 500 mg bid × 1–3 days; other fluoroquinolones are probably equally effective, especially ofloxacin, levofloxacin, or norfloxacin.

Vaccines are often required or recommended for travel, and recommendations are made in Table 7. The general rule is that HIV-infected persons cannot receive live virus vaccines. If there is anticipated exposure to typhoid fever, the inactivated injected

Table 7. Vaccines for Travel

Disease	Acceptable	Avoid	Comment
Polio	eIPV	Oral polio	Close contacts should also receive eIPV
Hepatitis A	—	HAV vaccine	Live virus vaccine; use gammaglobulin
Typhoid	Typhim Vi	Ty21a (Vivotif)	Inactivated parenteral vaccine is also acceptable
Japanese B encephalitis	JBE vaccine	—	
Yellow fever	—	Vaccine—avoid with CD4 < 200	Advise patient of risk and risk prevention (mosquito) and provide waiver
Meningitis	Meningo-cocceal vaccine	—	Use when indicated by travel to meningitis belt of Africa or when indicated by outbreaks

vaccine is recommended rather than the live vaccine form that is given by mouth. For yellow fever, the only vaccine is a live virus vaccine that has uncertain safety in people with HIV infection; if there is travel to an area with yellow fever, it may be necessary to obtain a letter indicating vaccination waiver, and there must be extra caution in avoiding mosquito bites. Killed vaccines are not a problem; these include the standard diphtheria-tetanus, rabies, meningococcal vaccines, and Japanese encephalitis vaccines.

Travelers must be aware about the types of infectious diseases that may pose particular risks in various areas. When malaria prophylaxis is indicated, there is concern about drug interactions between mefloquine and protease inhibitors. Preferred alternative for the patient taking HAART are doxycycline, chloroquine, atovaquones and proquainil. Many developing countries have high rates of tuberculosis, and HIV-infected persons are more than 100 times more likely to get this infection than persons without HIV infection. Many areas pose a risk for malaria, and the standard precautions include avoidance of insect bites and certain preventive drugs that should not be a problem for HIV-infected persons. Visceral leishmaniasis (kala azar) is a disease transmitted by sandflies in many tropical countries that can be a major problem in patients with HIV infection. This includes South and Central America (New World) and Asia, Africa, and Southern Europe (Old World). The same applies to *Penicillium marneffei* in the Far East: Thailand, Hong Kong, China, Vietnam, Indonesia (Lancet 1994;344:110).

Despite these concerns, there is relatively little to support the claim that travel, even in late stages of HIV infection, is too dangerous owing to exposures in other countries if simple precautions are taken.

Occupational Risks.   The major occupational risks to persons with HIV infection are in health care and child care and occupations that require animal contact. In the health care field, the major risk is TB exposure; this might also apply to employment in correctional facilities, shelters for the homeless, and volunteers for these sites. The specific risk depends to a large extent on the activities of the worker/volunteer and the prevalence of TB in the community. The major risk to providers of child care are *Cryptosporidium* and, to a lesser extent, *Cytomegalovirus,* hepatitis A, and giardiasis. The risk may be substantially reduced simply by good hygiene. Occupations requiring animal contact include veterinary work and employment in farms, slaughterhouses, or pet stores. The major risks are for *Cryptosporidium, Toxoplasma, Salmonella, Campylobacter,* and *Bartonella.* There is not good evidence that these occupations are sufficiently risky to avoid continued employment; the recommendation is to be aware of the risk and use appropriate precautions.

Most Common Presentations

Major diagnostic considerations based on physical findings are summarized in Table 8.

Laboratory Testing

The usual laboratory tests performed with initial evaluation are designed to (*a*) ensure confirmation of HIV infection; (*b*) stage the disease; (*c*) identify latent pathogens that will influence subsequent strategies for treatment and prophylaxis; and (*d*) determine general health status. Specific guidelines are summarized in Table 9.

HIV Serology.   Guidelines for HIV serology in terms of indications, interpretation, and use of alternative tests are summarized in Chapter 1. It is emphasized that 25–35% of patients

Table 8. Major Diagnostic Considerations by Organ System[a]

Conditions	CD4 >300/mm³	CD4 <200/mm³
Lymphadenopathy	PGL (syphilis, lymphoma, KS, TB)	PGL (CMV, TB, KS, MA)
Eye (fundi)		
Exudate + hemorrhage		CMV retinitis
Cotton wool spots	HIV retinopathy	HIV retinopathy
Oral		
White patches	Thrush, OHL	Thrush, OHL
Ulcers	HSV, aphthous ulcers	HSV, aphthous ulcers, CMV
Red-purple nodular lesions	KS	KS
Esophagus (dysphagia)		*Candida*, CMV, aphthous ulcers (HSV)
Abdomen		
Diarrhea	*Salmonella, C. difficile, Campylobacter, Shigella,* viral agents, cryptosporidiosis, *E. coli*	*Cryptosporidium*, microsporidia, MA, CMV, adverse drug reaction, *C. difficile*, AIDS enteropathy (small bowel overgrowth, histoplasmosis, Isospora, cyclospora, lymphoma)
Hepatomegaly and/or abnormal LFTs	Hepatitis (usually HBV or HCV), adverse drug reaction	Hepatitis (HBV or HCV), CMV, MA, lactic acidosis, lymphoma, HIV, fatty liver secondary to malnutrition; cholangiopathy-*Cryptosporidium*, CMV, idiopathic, (microsporidia)
Splenomegaly	HIV	Lymphoma, MA, histoplasmosis, HIV, cirrhosis

Skin		
Purple-black nodular lesions	KS (bacillary angiomatosis, prurigo nodularis)	KS (bacillary angiomatosis, prurigo nodularis)
Vesicles	Herpes simplex, herpes zoster	Herpes simplex, herpes zoster (CMV)
Maculopapular lesions	Adverse drug reaction, syphilis	Adverse drug reaction, syphilis
Plaques, scaling lesions	Seborrhea (psoriasis, eczema)	Seborrhea (psoriasis, eczema)
Umbilicated papules	Molluscum	Molluscum (cryptococcus)
Petechiae, purpura	ITP	ITP
Nodules		Cryptococcus, histoplasmosis, pruritis nodularis
Lungs		
Pneumonia	*S. pneumoniae,* (*H. influenzae,* TB, aspiration, atypical agents)	PCP, bacterial infections (TB, MA, KS, CMV, cryptococcus, histoplasmosis, lymphocytic interstitial pneumonia)
Cavity, nodules	TB (*S. aureus* with IV drug users)	TB (cryptococcus, nocardia, KS, lymphoma, MA, *M. kansasii,* atypical PCP, *Rhodococcus, Aspergillus*)
Neurological		
Aseptic meningitis	Neurosyphilis, viral	Cryptococcus
Chronic meningitis	Tuberculosis, neurosyphilis	Cryptococcus, tuberculosis, neurosyphilis
Dementia	Trauma, tumor, depression, hypothyroid	HIV-associated dementia
Constitutional symptoms (FUO, weight loss, etc.)	Lymphoma, TB	MA, CMV, histoplasmosis, HIV, cryptococcosis, PCP, lymphoma

[a] CMV, cytomegalovirus; FUO, fever of unknown origin; PCP, *P. carinii* pneumonia; MA, *M. avium;* TB, tuberculosis; OHL, oral hairy leukoplakia; PGL, peripheral generalized lymphadenopathy; HSV, herpes simplex virus; ADC, AIDS dementia complex.
[b] Conditions in parentheses indicate less likely diagnoses.

Table 9. Routine Laboratory Tests in Patients with HIV Infection (see DHHS Guidelines: MMWR 1998;47(RR-3):38)

Test	Cost	Frequency	Comment
HIV serology	Average $40	Once	• Repeat test for patients who have no identified risks, no confirmed test if plasma HIV RNA is negative or not done
CBC	$6–8	Every 3–6 mo	• Repeat more frequently with marrow suppression
CD4 count	$40–150	Every 3–6 mo	• Standard method to monitor immunocompetency • Routine testing is unnecessary for untreated patients with CD4 count <50/mm^3 • Outlier results should be confirmed owing to large variations in test results
Plasma HIV RNA	$80–240	Every 3–4 mo and 4–8 wk after new therapy	• Standard method to evaluate prognosis and response to therapy • Recommendation is baseline tests × 2 separated by ≥2 wk; with initiation of treatment or change in treatment. Test should be repeated at 4–8 wk to determine initial response (alpha slope) and at 4–6 mo to determine maximal effect (beta slope) • Testing should be done using same lab, same technique, at a time of clinical stability, and ≥1 mo from immunizations
Serum chemistries	$10–15	Annual or more frequent	• Major interest is hepatic function test owing to high rates of chronic hepatitis • Monitoring more frequently with use of nephrotoxic or hepatotoxic drugs including NNRTIs and protease inhibitors (PIs)
Anti-HBc	$10–15	Once in candidates for HBV vaccine	• Candidate for HBV vaccine

Test	Cost	Frequency	Comments
Anti-HCV and HBsAg	$40–60	Once in patient with unexplained abnormal LFTs	
Toxoplasma IgG	$12–15	Once (see comments)	• Screen all patients and repeat in seronegatives if 1) CD4 count <100/mm^3 and patient does not take TMP-SMX prophylaxis and 2) symptoms suggesting toxoplasmosis
PPD	$1	Annually	• Indicated if no history of positive PPD or treatment of TB • Repeat annually if high risk of TB and with exposure
Chest x-ray	$40–100	See comment	• Commonly advocated at baseline but prior study of 1065 HIV-infected patients showed virtually no useful information (Arch Intern Med 1996;156:191) • Indicated in patients with positive PPD, history of chest disease, or pulmonary symptoms
Pap smear	$25–40	Baseline, 6 mo, then annually	• Repeat results reported as inadequate • Refer to gynecologist for atypia or greater on the Bethesda score
CMV serology	$10–15	See comment	• Advocated for detection of latent CMV in low-risk patients to 1) permit counseling for CMV prevention (same as HIV), 2) assist in differential diagnosis of possible CMV disease, and 3) guide use of CMV-antibody negative blood or leukocyte-reduced blood products
VDRL or RPR	$5–16	Annually in sexually active patients	• Positives must have FTA confirmation: Up to 6% of HIV-infected patients have false-positive screening tests (CID 1994;19:1040; Am J Med 1995;99:55)
Fasting lipid profile and glucose	$15–25	Baseline and at 3–6 mo in patients given HAART	• Purpose is to evaluate risk for atherosclerosis and diabetes as complications of treatment with protease inhibitors and possibly with NNRTIs • Frequency of testing during therapy depends on results at 3–6 mo and additional risks

CBC, complete blood count; CMV, cytomegalovirus; DHHS, Department of Health and Human Services; HAART, highly active antiretroviral therapy; HBV, hepatitis B vaccine; LFTs, liver function tests; NNRTIs, nonnucleoside reverse transcriptase inhibitors; Pap, Papanicolaou; PIs, protease inhibitors; PPD, purified protein derivative; RPR, rapid plasma reagin; VDRL, Venereal Disease Research Laboratory.

with HIV infection in the US are unaware of their infection. The CDC recommends serologic testing for all patients who are sexually active (Clin Infect Dis 2004;38:104). The rapid test should notably facilitate this objective. AIDS-defining complication and CD4 counts may serve as a surrogate marker for advanced HIV infection in patients with possible HIV-related complications when serology results are delayed or serology is refused. The CBC can be used to detect lymphopenia ($<1000/mm^3$), which is supportive. A CD4 count is more specific because relatively few common conditions in medicine other than HIV cause severe depletion of CD4 cells, although acute steroid therapy may do this. Other causes of reduced CD4 counts include sarcoid, radiation, atopic dermatitis, collagen-vascular diseases, lymphoma, Sjögen's syndrome, and idiopathic CD4 lymphopenia (NEJM 1993;328:373, 380, 386; CID 2002;38:E125).

CD4 Cell Count.   Mean levels in healthy controls for most laboratories are $800–1050/mm^3$, with a range representing two standard deviations of about $450–1400/mm^3$ (Ann Intern Med 1993;119:55). There is substantial variation in the test results owing to technology, diurnal variations, and possible influence of intercurrent illnesses. Diurnal variations show lowest levels at 12:30 PM and peak values at 8:30 PM. The average diurnal change in HIV-infected persons with counts of 200–500 is $60/mm^3$ (J AIDS 1990;3:144). Marked laboratory variations reflect the fact that the count represents the product of three variables: White blood cell count, percent lymphocytes, and percent lymphocytes that bear the CD4 receptor. High-quality laboratories participating in AIDS Clinical Treatment Group (ACTG) trials showed the average within-subject coefficient of variation was 25% (JID 1994;169:28). A comparison of four labs performing tests on 24 patients showed the average difference between high and low values was $108/mm^3$; 14 of the 24 had results that would lead to different therapeutic decisions (CID 1995;21: 1121). The 95% confidence limits indicate that the reporting range for a value of $500/mm^3$ is $297–841/mm^3$. Standards for quality assurance have recently been published by the CDC (MMWR 1997;46[RR-2]). Methods to reduce variations are to use the same laboratory, sample patients at times of clinical stability, and maintain consistency in the time of blood draws. Some clinicians prefer the CD4 percent because this reduces variation to one measurement (J AIDS 1989;2:114). Corresponding CD4 cell counts follow:

CD4 Cell Count	%CD4
>500/mm^3	>29
200–500/mm^3	14–28
<200/mm^3	<14

Deceptively high CD4 counts may be seen with a splenectomy or concurrent HTLV-1 infection. Splenectomy results in a rapid sustained increase in the CD4 count; the CD4 percentage is a better indicator of immune function (Arch Surg 1998;133:25; Clin Infect Dis 1995;20:768). HTLV-1 infection is uncommon in the U.S. HTLV-2 is far more common and occurs in association with injection drug use and commercial sex work (N Engl J Med 1990;326:375). Unfortunately, most laboratories do not distinguish HTLV-1 and HTLV-2. With HTLV-1, the CD4 counts are artificially elevated 80–180% (JAMA 1994;271:353). Factors that have little or no influence on CD4 counts are stress, exercise, sex, pregnancy, and risk category.

Quantitative HIV RNA. Plasma HIV RNA level measurement (viral load) is a standard method to evaluate risk of progression and response to therapy. The best data for its prognostic value are from the MACS, which is a prospective longitudinal study of HIV infection in gay men that was initiated in 1984. Results with sampling every 6 mo in a large cohort of essentially untreated men (Table 10) (Ann Internal Med 1997;126:946). The MACS data show that VL is a significant predictor of progression that is independent of the CD4, but its value is greatest in early stage disease because it drives the CD4 slope (Table 11). In late stage disease the CD4 count is a much stronger predictor of outcome in terms of opportunistic infections, wasting, morbidity and death (Lancet 2002;360:119). The goal of therapy is "no detectable virus" using a threshold 400–500 copies/mL or a threshold of 20–50 copies/mL; it is expected that commercially available tests in the future will detect 2–5 copies/mL.

There are three commercially available methods to measure viral load that are summarized in Table 10. The reproducibility

Table 10. Quantitative HIV RNA

	Roche* 800-526-1247	Bayer (Formerly Chiron) 800-434-2447	Organon 800-682-2666 ×5
Technique	RT-PCR	bDNA	NASBA
Dynamic range	Amplicor HIV-1 1.0 and 1.5 400–750,000 copies/mL Ultrasensitive: 40–75,000 copies/mL	Version 3.0 (preferred): 100–500,000 copies/ mL Version 2.0: 500–500,000 copies/ mL	Nuclisens HIV-1 QT: 176–3,500,000 copies/mL depending on volume
Subtypes quantitated	Version 1.0-B only Version 1.5-A–G	A–H	A–G
Specimen volume	Amplicor 1.0: 0.2 mL Ultrasensitive: 0.5 mL	1 mL	10 μL–2 mL
Tubes	EDTA (lavender top)	EDTA (lavender top)	EDTA, heparin, whole blood, body fluid, semen, tissue, etc.
Relative merits	Amplicor 1.0 quantitate only subtype B; other subtypes are low. Version 1.5 quantitates subgroups A–G	Technician demand is less Quantitates subtypes A–H	Will quantitate HIV in many body fluids and tissue Quantitates subtypes A–G

* Amplicor version 1.0 is to be phased out.

Table 11. Viral Burden Analysis

Viral Burden (copies/mL)*	No. of Patients	Relative Hazard		Median Survival (yr)	CD4 Slope
		AIDS	Death		
<500	112	1.0	1.0	>10	−36
500–3,000	229	2.4	2.8	>10	−45
3,000–10,000	347	4.4	5.0	>10	−55
10,000–30,000	357	7.6	9.9	7.5	−65
>30,000	386	13	18.5	4.4	−76

* MACS data (Ann Intern Med 1997;126:946).

of these tests is about 0.3 $\log_{10}$ copies/mL or about 2-fold. Results with RT-PCR are approximately the same as with bDNA (J Clin Microbiol 2000;38:2837); values for the Nuclisens assay appear comparable as well, but the correlation is less well studied (JCM 2000;38:3882; JCM 2000;38:3837). Plasma HIV RNA levels are about 2-fold lower in women compared with men for the same prognosis in terms of CD4 count, AIDS defining complications, or death; these differences disappear with progression to later stages (Lancet 1998;352:1510; NEJM 2001;344:720; CID 2002;35:313).

Resistance Testing. This is an in vitro method to measure susceptibility of HIV strains to antiretroviral agents. There are two basic methods that have different merits.

Genotypic assays. Genotypic assays measure mutations on the reverse transcriptase (RT) or protease (P) gene. Mutations are reported for each gene using a letter-number-letter standard in which the first letter indicates the amino acid at the designated codon in wild-type virus; the number is the codon, and the second letter indicates the substituted amino acid (Table 12) (Topics in HIV Med 2002;5:21). Resistance mutations are classified as "major" or "minor" for protease inhibitors. This distinction has been discontinued for mutations on the RT gene.

Phenotypic assays. Phenotypic assays are offered by Virco and ViroLogic. These are more analogous to conventional antibacterial sensitivity tests with results reported as the -fold increase in resistance compared with wild-type virus. The levels selected to define resistance were formerly quite arbitrary, usually 1.7-, 4-, or 10-fold higher than wild-type virus, meaning the

Table 12. Codon Mutations that Confer Resistance to Antiretroviral Agents
(Updates Available at www.iasusa.org)

PI	Major	Minor
IDV	46L, 82AFT, 84V	10IRV, 20MR, 24I, 32I, 36I, 54V, 71VI, 73SA, 71I, 90M
NFV	30N, 90M	10FI, 36I, 46IL, 71VI, 77I, 82AFTS, 84V, 88DS
RTV	82AFTS, 84V	10FIRV, 20MR, 32I, 33F, 36I, 46IL, 54VL, 71VT, 77I, 90M
SQV	48V, 90M	10IRV, 54VL, 71VT, 73S, 77I, 82A, 84V
APV/FPV	50V, 84V	10FIRV, 32I, 46IL, 47V, 54VM, 73S, 90M
LPV/r	—	10FIRV, 20MR, 24I, 31I, 33F, 46IL, 47VA, 50V, 53I, 54VLAMTS, 71VT, 73S, 82AFTS, 84V, 90
ATV	50L	10IFV, 20RMI, 24I, 32I, 33I, FV, 36ILV, 46I, 48V, 54V, 71V, 73CSTA, 82A, 84V, 88S, 90M
TPV	33I, 82AFLT, 84V, 90M	10IV, 20MLT, 46I, 54V
Multi PI	46IL, 82AFTS, 84VAC, 90M	

Agent	Resistance Mutations
Nucleosides/Nucleotides	
AZT	41 L, 44 D, 67 N, 70 R, 118 I, 210 W, 215 YF, 219 Q
d4T	41 L, 44 D, 65 R, 67 N, 70 R, 118 I, 210 W, 215 YF, 219 QE
3 TC	44 D, 65 R, 118 I, 184 VI
FTC	65 R, 184 VI
ddC	65 R, 69 D, 74 V, 184 V
ddI	65 R, 74 V
ABC	65 R, 74 V, 115 F, 184 V
TDF	65 R
Multi-151	62 V, 75 I, 77 L, 116 Y, 151 M
Multi-69	41 L, 62 V, 67 N, 69 Insertion, 70 R, 210 W, 215 YF, 219 QE
Multi-TAMs	41 L, 44 D, 67 N, 70 R, 118 I, 210 W, 215 YF, 219 QE
Non-Nucleoside RT Inhibitors	
NVP	100 I, 103 N, 106 AM, 108 I, 181 CI, 188 CLH, 190A
DLV	103 N, 106 M, 181 C, 188 L, 236 L
EFV	101 I, 103 N, 106 M, 108 I, 181 CI, 188 L, 190 SA, 225 H
Multi-1	103 N, 106 M, 188 I
Multi-2	100 I, 106 A, 181 CI, 190 SA, 230 L

* Top HIV Med 2003;11:215.

test strain was 1.7-, 4-, or 10-fold more resistant than wild-type virus for any specific drug. The present reporting system uses standardized thresholds for each drug based on clinical trial experience and other data (JID 2001;183:401) but does not account for RTV-boosted PIs.

Virtual phenotype.   This is a combination of both methods using the genotypic assay to define mutations, which is then matched with the phenotype of previously tested strains that have the same mutational pattern.

Relative merits of assays.   There are two limitations for both types of assays. 1) They measure only the dominant HIV species; variants that account for <20% of the total viral population tested are not tested. The implication is that resistant strains representing minority species and/or present only in sequestered sites will not be detected. Thus, results are most accurate in defining activity vs. drugs given at the time of testing. 2) Neither assay can be performed on specimens with viral loads <500–1000 copies/mL. 3) A third limitation is the diffi-

Table 13. Comparison of Genotypic and Phenotypic Assays to Detect HIV Resistance

	Genotypic Assay	Phenotypic Assay
Availability	Widely available	Less readily available
Cost	$360–$480/test for RT and P gene	$800–$1000
Turnaround time	7–14 days	14–21 days
Viral load required	>1000 copies/mL	>500–1000 copies/mL
Interpretation	Requires knowledge of effect of each mutational change	More analogous to in vitro sensitivity tests for bacteria
	Results are confounded by incomplete knowledge of resistance mutations	Thresholds to define sensitivity do not account for RTV-boosted PI levels
	May fail to correlate with phenotypic resistance	Measures total effect
	Very reproducible	Very reproducible
		Two suppliers (ViroLogic and Virco): Both validated and never compared

culty in interpreting results with both assays. Relative merits of the tests are summarized in Table 13 (J AIDS 2001;26:53).

Indications.   Resistance testing is advocated according to virtually all guidelines, including the DHHS guidelines (www.hivatis.org). The only exception is in areas where such testing is not available.

Recommendations.   Virologic failure—to facilitate the selection of the next regimen and preserve options. This is the major category in which there is a consensus agreement about the use of resistance tests. Most authorities also advocate resistance tests for patients with acute HIV. This will facilitate drug selection if antiretroviral therapy is given. Even without early therapy, this information may be useful at a later time because it should reveal the resistance profile of the transmitted strain. When used for early therapy, these results should not delay antiretroviral therapy (BMJ 2001;322:1087).

Practical issues.   Resistance testing is sometimes advocated for drug selection in the initial treatment of chronically infected patients but may be misleading since wild-type virus usually dominates. Nevertheless, some resistance mutations persist for at least 1 year or longer. Some test at baseline because it may reveal drugs to avoid. An alternative strategy is to give therapy for 2–4 wk to exert the pressure that would reveal resistance mutations in minor strains at baseline. In general, patients should be tested while they are receiving the drug, but the duration of time off therapy that retains validity is difficult to define and probably varies with drug, viral load, and other factors. When treatment is stopped, it is usually 2–6 wk before there is resolution of resistance mutations, and some persist for much longer. It can consequently be argued that the best time for testing is while the failing regimen is given, but delays of weeks and possibly longer may still be valid. With the patient who has had multiple regimens, resistance testing will not generally reveal relevant information about drugs other than the most recent regimen except for class cross-reactions. Drug history and prior sensitivity test results are critical here.

Syphilis Serology.   Screening tests (VDRL or RPR) should be performed with the initial evaluation and repeated annually in patients who are sexually active. False-negative and false-positive tests have been reported in patients with HIV infection (JID 1990;162:862; JID 1992;165:1020; AIDS 1991;5:419), but these are rare (Ann Intern Med 1990;113:872). Patients with a positive screening test should have a confirmatory fluorescent treponemal antibody absorption test.

Serum Chemistry Panel.   The screen should include tests of liver function (bilirubin, transaminase levels, alkaline phosphatase), renal function, and glucose.

Hepatitis B Serology.   HBsAg is tested to determine if the patient has chronic hepatitis caused by HBV; many such patients are candidates for therapy with interferon, lamivudine, tenofovir, or emtricitabine. This information will also influence how these three nucleosides/nucleotides are used for treating HIV. Anti-HBc or anti-HBs is measured to determine candidates for HBV vaccine. Patients with HIV have a CD4 cell count dependent response—only 50–70% with CD4 counts below $200/mm^3$ develop antibody levels of >10 units/mL after three doses; these patients are candidates for one additional three dose series.

Hepatitis C.   About 90% of long-term injection drug users have positive HCV serology, and about 85% of these are chronic carriers (MMWR 1998;47[RR-19]). Seroprevalence of HCV in the general population in the United States is 1.8% for adults. Seroprevalence among patients with HIV is about 30% but varies with risk category depending largely on the number with injection drug use. HCV serology should be obtained in all HIV-infected patients. The usual screening test is EIA for anti-HCV which shows a sensitivity of >99% in immunocompetent patients, but shows more frequent false negatives with HIV co-infections (JAIDS 2002;31:154). The qualitative HCV RNA test is positive in these cases. HCV infected patients who are candidates for therapy should be evaluated with quantitative HCV RNA genotypic analysis, and liver biopsy (see National Institutes of Health [NIH] Consensus Report #60 issued 8/20/02 on Management of Hepatitis C).

Toxoplasmosis Serology.   IgG for *T. gondii* is advocated 1) at the initial screen to determine latent infection, 2) in previously seronegative or untested patients who become candidates for toxoplasmosis prophylaxis using agents other than TMP-SMX (given for PCP prophylaxis) because of a CD4 count of $<100/mm^3$, and 3) in previously seronegative or untested patients who have possible central nervous system (CNS) toxoplasmosis. Seroprevalence for adults in the U.S. is 10–11% in HIV infected adults in the United States (JAIDS 1993;6:414; CID 2002;35:1414). Seroprevalence in Latin America, Europe, Asia, and Africa is 30–75% (JID 1988;157:1; Lancet 2004;363:1965). The sensitivity of the test in patients with CNS toxoplasmosis is 90–100%.

Cytomegalovirus Serology.   This is sometimes advocated with initial evaluation to detect latent CMV infection in patients with a low risk of harboring CMV (MMWR 2002;51:RR-8:17). Seroprevalence of CMV in healthy adults in the United States is 50–70%; it is >90% in gay men, IDUs, and hemophiliacs. Other tests for CMV include culture PCR assays and NASBA early antigen assay; none of these has proved useful for predicting CMV disease (J Clin Micro 2000;38:563).

PPD Skin Test.   The CDC recommends routine testing with PPD (using the standard Mantoux test) 5TU units with interpretation at 48–72 hr by a health care professional. This should be performed at baseline in all persons with HIV infection who do not have a history of TB or of a prior positive test. It should be repeated annually in high-risk patients. Induration of >5 mm constitutes a positive result (MMWR 2002;51:RR-6). A prospective study of 1130 HIV-infected persons followed a median of 53 mo showed the rate of active TB was 0.5/100 in those who remained PPD negative compared with 3.2/100 in those with baseline positive PPD tests and 4.7/100 in those who seroconverted (Ann Intern Med 1997;126:123). Anergy testing is not recommended because of lack of standardization of reagents and inconsistent results with repeat tests in HIV-infected patients (Arch Intern Med 1993;155:2111).

Pap Smear.   The CDC recommends a gynecologic evaluation with pelvic examination and Pap smear in women with HIV infection at initial evaluation, a repeat Pap smear 6 mo later, and then annually if results are normal (MMWR 1990;39:

Table 14. Management of Abnormal Pap Smear Test Results: Recommendations of the Agency for Health Care Policy and Research and National Cancer Institute (JAMA 2002;287:211)

Results	Action
Inadequate	Repeat
Inflammation	Evaluate for infection, treat, and repeat Pap smear in 2–3 mo
Atypia (ASCUS) • ACS-US (undetermined significance)* • ACS-H (cannot exclude HSIL)*	Repeat Pap smear every 4–6 mo × 2 yr to achieve three consecutive negative smears or colposcopy (see footnote)
Low-grade squamous intraepithelial lesion (LGSIL or LSIL) (CIN 1)	Colposcopy and biopsy or follow-up Pap smear every 4–6 mo; consider repeat colposcopy annually
High-grade squamous intraepithelial lesions (HGSIL or HSIL) (CIN 2 or 3)	Colposcopy and biopsy; treat with loop excision or conization
Invasive carcinoma	Refer to gynecologic oncologist for surgery or radiation

* ACS-H/ACS-US are new designations (JAMA 2002;287:211). Most gynecologists recommend evaluation of any abnormality in women with HIV.

47). Current recommendations for managing results are shown in Table 14.

Chest X-Ray. A chest x-ray is recommended for detection of asymptomatic TB and also as a baseline test for patients who have high rates of pulmonary disease. A review of screening chest x-rays in 1065 HIV-infected persons at 0-, 3-, 6-, and 12-mo intervals showed only 2% were abnormal, and this technique detected only 11 of 55 patients who developed pulmonary complications within 2 mo of the x-ray (Arch Intern Med 1996;156: 191). The yield was also low in groups at high risk for TB and those with low CD4 counts. The authors concluded that chest x-rays as a screening test in asymptomatic HIV-infected persons with a negative PPD are unwarranted.

Lipid Profile. Patients who are candidates for HAART should have a baseline analysis of cholesterol (HDL and LDL), fasting triglycerides, and fasting blood glucose. This should be repeated about 3–6 mo after initiating a regimen containing a protease inhibitor or an NNRTI. The test should be repeated annually or more frequently if there are abnormal results and in some high-risk patients. Most patients who have blood lipid abnormalities or insulin resistance will show abnormal test results within 3–6 mo. These results become the database for decisions regarding changes in treatment or introduction of methods to prevent atherosclerosis using the National Cholesterol Education guidelines (see Table 38). Abnormal blood glucose levels should be managed according to guidelines for diabetic control.

Glucose-6-Phosphate Dehydrogenase Level.   Glucose-6-phosphate dehydrogenase (G-6-PD) deficiency is a genetic disease that predisposes to hemolytic anemia after exposure to oxidant drugs. There are more than 300 variants that are inherited on the X chromosome. The most common form is GdA, which is found in 10% of black males and 1–2% of black females; the most serious form is GdMED, which is found predominantly in males from the Mediterranean area (Italians, Greeks, Sephardic Jews, Arabs) and males from India and Southeast Asia. In most cases, the hemolysis is mild and self-limited because only the older red cells are involved and the bone marrow can compensate. The most important exception is GdMED, which may cause life-threatening hemolysis. The severity of anemia also depends on concentration of the drug in the red cells and the oxidant potential; the most likely offending agents used in patients with HIV infection are dapsone and primaquine and less likely are sulfonamides. During hemolysis, G-6-PD levels are usually normal because the susceptible red cells have been destroyed so that testing must be delayed for about 1 mo after a drug holiday. Methemoglobin levels will be elevated. Options for testing are to 1) obtain this test at baseline; 2) screen patients at high risk (African-American males and males of Mediterranean descent); 3) delay testing until oxidant drugs are indicated; or 4) delay until hemolysis is suspected (with measurement of methemoglobin acutely and level of G-6-PD after a drug holiday). Most patients with low levels tolerate oxidant drugs well; it would be a mistake to consider, for example, TMP-SMX or dapsone to be absolutely contraindicated in an African-American male with an abnormally low G-6-PD level.

General Health Screens

Test	Age	Frequency
Mammogram	Female >40 yr	Annual
Pap Smear	All	Baseline, 6 mo, then annually
Colonoscopy	>50 yr	Every 5–6 yr
Occult blood—stool	>50 yr	
PSA	>50 yr	Repeat periodically

5—Prevention: Opportunistic Infections
USPHS/IDSA Guidelines (MMWR 1999; 48(RR-10))

The U.S. Public Health Service and the Infectious Diseases Society of America provided guidelines on strategies to reduce the frequency of opportunistic infections that were originally published in 1995 (MMWR 1995;44(RR-8); CID 1995;21(Suppl 1)), revised in 1997 (Ann Intern Med 1997;127:939) and re-revised in 2001 (MMWR 2002;51:RR-6). The most recent recommendations are presented in the following tables.

Table 15: Prevention of Opportunistic Infections: Antimicrobial Prophylaxis

Table 16: Recommendations for Primary and Secondary Opportunistic Infection Prophylaxis during Pregnancy

Table 17: Recommendations for Vaccines in HIV-Infected Patients

Table 15. Prevention of Opportunistic Infections: Antimicrobial Prophylaxis
Recommendation of USPHS/IDSA (MMWR 2002;51(RR-6))

Disease	Indications: Start and Stop*	Preferred Regimen (drug cost/mo)	Comment/Alternative/Stopping recs (www.hivatis.org 1/3/03)
STRONGLY RECOMMENDED AS STANDARD OF CARE			
TB (latent) (MMWR 2000;47;RR-6; MMWR 2001;50:773)	PPD + (≥5 mm induration) Prior positive PPD without prior INH prophylaxis High-risk exposure	INH 300 mg/day + pyridoxine 50 mg/d ≥270 doses, 9 mo or up to 12 mo with interruptions ($2.00/mo) INH 900 mg + pyridoxine 100 mg 2–3/wk with DOT ≥76 doses, 9 mo or up to 12 mo with interruptions ($0.60/mo) INH resistant strain: Rifampin 600 mg/day × 4 mo or Rifabutin (see doses Table 46) × 4 mo Multiply resistant: Fluoroquinolone + PZA or ethambutol + PZA	Rifampin 600 mg/day + pyrazinamide 20 mg/kg/day with ≥60 doses × 2 mo or up to 3 mo with interruptions ($268/mo)** Risk of severe hepatotoxicity—use only with patients unlikely to complete 9-month INH course plus no prior NIH associated hepatotoxicity or prior liver disease Monitor LTs at baseline, 2, 4, and 6 wk and prescribe only a 2-wk supply to assure observations • Alternative (INH resistance or toxicity): Rifampin 600 mg/d × 4 mo • Alternative for patient receiving PI or NNRTI who needs to take a rifamycin (see rifampin and rifabutin drug interactions Table 42) • Contact with INH-resistant strain: Rifamycin + pyrazinamide × 2 mo as noted previously

Table 15. (continued)

Disease	Indications: Start and Stop*	Preferred Regimen (cost/mo)	Comment/Alternative
P. carinii pneumonia	*Start prophylaxis:* Prior PCP CD4 <200/mm³ Thrush or FUO *Stop prophylaxis:* Primary* prophylaxis: when CD4 >200/ mm³ × 3 mo Secondary prophylaxis: when CD4 >200 × 3 mo	TMP-SMX 1 DS/d ($6/mo) or 1 SS/day	• *Alternatives:* TMP-SMX 1 DS 3 day/wk; dapsone 100 mg/day ($6/mo); regimens for toxoplasmosis prophylaxis (see below), aerosolized pentamidine 300 mg/mo ($120/mo + administration costs) or atovaquone 750 mg bid with meals ($980/mo) • Safety of discontinuation of prophylaxis is well confirmed (NEJM 2001;344:159; NEJM 2001; 344:168; CID 2001;33:1901)
Toxoplasmosis	*Start prophylaxis:* CD4 <100/mm³ *plus* positive serology (IgG) *Stop prophylaxis:* Primary prophylaxis*: when CD4 >200/ mm³ × 3 mo Secondary prophylaxis*: when CD4 >200 × ≥6 mo, asymptomatic & completed initial Rx	TMP-SMX 1 DS/day ($6/mo)	• *Alternatives:* in patients with TMP-SMX intolerance: Dapsone 50 mg/day + pyrimethamine 50 mg/wk + leucovorin 25 mg/wk ($35/mo) or dapsone 200 mg/wk + pyrimethamine 75 mg/wk + leucovorin 25 mg/wk ($40/mo) or atovaquone 1500 mg/day ± pyrimethamine 25 mg qd + leucovorin 10 mg/day ($2000/ mo) • Immune reconstitution: Safety of discontinuation of secondary prophylaxis is established (Ann Intern Med 2002;137:239)

M. avium complex	*Start prophylaxis:* CD4 <50/mm³ *Stop prophylaxis:* Primary prophylaxis: when CD4 >100/ mm³ × 3 mo Secondary prophylaxis: when CD4 >100 × ≥6 mo + 12 mo Rx + asymptomatic	Clarithromycin 500 mg bid ($240/mo) Azithromycin 1200 mg 1 ×/wk ($136/mo)

- *Alternatives:* rifabutin 300 mg/ day ($330/mo) or rifabutin 300 mg/day + azithromycin 1200 mg q wk (see dose adjustments for rifabutin and for PI/NNRTIs under TB prophylaxis previous page) ($460/mo)
- A disadvantage of clarithromycin (which is the favored agent for treatment of established infection) is possible resistance
- Immune reconstitution: Data support discontinuation of primary prophylaxis (NEJM 2000; 342:1085; Ann Intern Med 2000; 133:493) and discontinuation of secondary prophylaxis: (AIDS 1999;13:1647; AIDS 2000;14:383; Ann Intern Med 2002;137:239)

Varicella	Exposure to chickenpox or zoster and no history of chickenpox or shingles or negative varicella-zoster virus (VZV) antibody	Varicella-zoster immune globulin (VZIG) 625 units (5 vials) IM ≤96 hr after exposure ($350)

- Acyclovir prophylaxis is no longer advocated because of no supporting data

Table 15. (continued)

Disease	Indications: Start and Stop*	Preferred Regimen (cost/mo)	Comment/Alternative
GENERALLY RECOMMENDED			
Streptococcus pneumoniae	CD4 count >200/mm³	Pneumococcal vaccine 0.5 mL IM × 1 ($11)	• Response is reduced in patients with CD4 counts <200/mm³ • Revaccination sometimes advocated with vaccination >5 yr ago or with immune reconstitution of CD4 to >200/mm³ • Evidence of efficacy is conflicting: One report shows 49% efficacy (Arch Intern Med 2000; 160:2633); another showed increased pneumococcal infection in vaccine recipients (Lancet 2000;355:2106)
Influenza	All patients	Influenza vaccine ($6)	• CDC guidelines are ambivalent. Favoring vaccination is one report showing influenza may have a worse course in HIV-infected patients and evidence that it works in this population. There is poor response in persons with CD4 counts <200/mm

| Hepatitis B | Negative anti-HBc screening test | HBV vaccine × three doses at 0, 1, and 6 mo ($161) | • Measure anti-HBsAg level at 1–6 mo after third dose; if <10 IU/mL repeat series
Alternative: none |

| Hepatitis A | Neg anti-HAV + risk (MSM, IDU) or chronic liver disease) | HAV vaccine × 2 at 0 & 6 mo ($60) | |

| | Selected high-risk patients | Amantadine 100 mg po bid ($36/mo)
Ramantadine 100 mg po bid ($132/mo)
Oselfamavir 75 mg po qd ($210/mo) | • Anti-influenza drugs: Use in high-risk patients with no vaccination or anticipated poor response (CD4 < 200). Amantadine has least cost, ramantadine is better-tolerated, and oselfamavir is active vs influenza B as well as A. |

* Primary prophylaxis means no prior disease with designated pathogen; secondary prophylaxis means prior disease with indicated pathogen.

Table 16. Antimicrobials Used for Treatment and Prevention of Opportunistic Infection in Pregnant Women with HIV Infection

Agent (FDA Category)*	Comment
Acyclovir Category B	Indicated for severe HSV and VZV infections. Use for prophylaxis is investigational
Albendazole Category C	Consider in 2nd and 3rd trimester for microsporidiosis
Amphotericin Category B	
Atovaquone Category C	Limited experience
Azithromycin Category B	Preferred agent for MAC
Cidofovir Category C	Teratogenic and embryotoxic in animals; risk in humans is unknown
Clarithromycin Category C	Teratogenic in rats; in human data—use alternative agent if possible
Clindamycin Category B	Safe in humans
Dapsone Category C	May risk kernicterus; limited human experience
Doxycycline Category D	Bone and tooth change in neonate—contraindicated
Ethambutol Category B	Teratogenic at high doses in mice; appears safe in humans
Famciclovir Category B	Limited human data—report exposures 1-888-669-6682
Fluconazole Category C	Structural defects in rats, skeletal abnormalities in 4 infants ater long exposure; single dose appears safe
Flucytosine Category C	Facial clefts etc. in rats and may be teratogenic; use after 1st trimester if needed
Fluoroquinolones Category C	Arthropathy in beagle dogs; no joint changes with > 200 first trimester exposures in humans
Foscarnet Category C	Skeletal abnormalities in rats; no data in humans—use for life-threatening CMV
Ganciclovir Category C	Embryotoxic and teratogenic in animals; case reports of safety in people
G-CSF Category C	Safe in rodents; case reports of safety in people
Interferon Category C	Possible risk of uterine growth retardation; > 30 cases in patients without toxicity
Isoniazid Category C	Possible hepatotoxicity; give pyridoxine to prevent neurotoxicity; give vitamin K at birth to prevent hemorrhagic disease
Itraconazole Category C	Teratogenic in rats; no defects noted with 156 first-trimester exposures
Metronidazole Category B	Large experience with first-trimester exposures shows no defects
Paromomycin Category C	Not absorbed—toxicity unlikely
Pentamidine Category C	Limited experience
Primaquine Category C	Theoretical risk of hemolytic anemia if infant is G6PD-deficient
Pyrazinamine Category C	Limited human experience
Pyrimethamine Category C	Teratogenic in rodents; limited data in humans
Ribavirin Category X	Multiple defects in rodents; contraindicated in first trimester
Rifabutin Category B	Appears safe; not teratogenic in rats

Table 16. (continued)

Agent (FDA Category)*	Comment
Rifampin Category C	Teratogenic in rats; not clearly teratogenic in humans; give vitamin K at birth
TMP-SMX Category C	Teratogenic in rats; possible congenital cardiac defects in people; Potential for kernicterus if used near delivery
Valacyclovir Category B	Limited experience in people, but probably similar to acyclovir
Valganciclovir Category C	Embryogenic and teratogenic in rodents; case reports of safe use in people.

* Category	Interpretation
A	Controlled studies show no risk. Adequate, well-controlled studies in pregnant women have failed to demonstrate risk to the fetus.
B	No evidence of risk in humans. Either animal findings show risk, but human findings do not, or, if no adequate human studies have been done, animal findings are negative.
C	Risk cannot be ruled out. Human studies are lacking, and animal studies are either positive for fetal risk, or lacking as well. However, potential benefits may justify the potential risk.
D	Positive evidence of risk. Investigational or postmarketing data show risk to the fetus. Nevertheles, potential benefits may outweigh the potential risk.
X	Contraindicated in pregnancy. Studies in animals or humans, or investigational or postmarketing reports, have shown fetal risk which clearly outweighs any possible benefit to the patient.

Table 17. Recommendations for Vaccines in HIV-Infected Patients[a]

Vaccine and Regimen (Cost[b])	Indication/Category	Comment
Routine vaccinations		
Pneumococcal vaccine 0.5 mL IM ($11.90)	All patients	Risk of S. pneumoniae bacteremia is increased 100-fold. Antigenic response is best when CD4 count is >200/mm^3. Revaccination consideration: >5 yr since prior vaccination or vaccination when CD4 < 200/mm^3 + immune reconstitution. Evidence of benefit is conflicting
Influenza vaccine 0.5 mL IM ($6)	All HIV patients in Oct–Dec	Risk of influenza (acquisition or severity) is increased. Prevention may avoid complicated diagnostic evaluation of flulike complaints. Vaccination may increase HIV viral burden, transiently, but significance is not considered important
	Alternatives in selected patients • Amantadine 100 mg po bid ($36/mo) • Ramantadine 100 mg po bid ($132/mo) • Oseltamavir 75 mg/d ($210/mo)	Amantadine (least cost), ramantadine (better-tolerated), and oseltamavir (active vs influenza B as well as A); these are advocated with high risk plus unvaccinated or anticipated poor response (CD4 < 200/mm^3)
Hepatitis B vaccine 3 IM doses at 0, 1, and 6 mo Recombivax 10 µg Engerix 20 µg ($55.78/dose or about $165 for the series)	All susceptible (negative anti-HBc test) patients	Screening test is anti-HBc or anti-HBs. Risk of becoming HBsAg carrier is increased with HIV infection. Measure antibody response at 1–6 mo after third-dose; nonresponders should receive repeat series

Hepatitis A 1-mL doses at 0 and 6 mo ($46/dose)	All susceptible (negative anti-HAV test) + chronic liver disease, MSM, or IDU	Risk of fulminant hepatitis with acute HAV in patients with chronic HCV infection About 30% of U.S. adult population has serologic evidence of prior HAV Many recommend HAV vaccination for all HIV-infected patients
Travel associated vaccines		
Oral polio—oral	Contraindicated	Live vaccine; eIPV preferred If inadvertently given to household contact, contact should be avoided for 1 mo
Inactivated polio (eIPV) 0.5 mL SC ($14.00)	Travel to developing countries for those without prior immunization	Preferred polio vaccine for HIV-infected persons and close contacts Polio has been eliminated from Western hemisphere
Yellow fever	Contraindicated	Live vaccine. With travel to endemic area advise patient of risk, instruct in control of mosquito exposure, and provide vaccination waiver letter
Japanese B encephalitis 1 mL SC ×3 at days 0, 7, and 30 ($200)	Travel >1 mo to epidemic area	Expensive and frequent side effects (not unique to HIV-infected persons)
Typhoid (ViCSP) 0.5 mL IM × 1 ($32.44)	Travel to risk area (Latin America, Asia, Africa)	Live attenuated Ty21 a vaccine (Vivotif) is contraindicated. ViCSP is more expensive and no more effective than the parenteral inactivated vaccine but causes fewer side effects and requires only one dose

Table 17. (continued)

Vaccine and Regimen (Cost[b])	Indication/Category	Comment
Typhoid inactivated vaccine 0.5 mL SC × 2 separated by 1 mo ($10.16/20 doses)	As previously	
Hepatitis A 1 mL adult formulation IM × 1 ≥14 days before travel ($60 single dose)	Travel to developing countries Gay men, injection drug users, chronic liver disease (see previous entry)	Havrix may be used in place of immune globulin Serologic tests show 30% of adults are protected by prior infection
Cholera vaccine	Not recommended	No longer recommended or required
Other Vaccines		
Haemophilus influenzae type B 0.5 mg IM × 1 ($20.46/dose)	Not recommended	Not recommended because most infections with *H. influenzae* in HIV-infected persons involve nontypable strains (JAMA 1992;268:3350)
Tetanus-diphtheria (Td) vaccine 0.5 mg IM q 10 yr ($2.40)	All adults—booster q 10 yr	HIV infection is not a contraindication
Measles, mumps, rubella (MMR) vaccine	Contraindicated	Live virus vaccine; one report of a serious reaction (MMWR 1995;43:959)

Varicella-zoster vaccine —	Contraindicated	Live virus vaccine; more than 90% of adults have serologic evidence of varicella infection; if HIV-infected person is seronegative—avoid contact with chickenpox and zoster
Vaccinia Standard 15-puncture method	Contraindicated for preemptive smallpox (no attack) Indicated if smallpox attack with exposure	Live virus vaccine Risk of progressive vaccinia due to depressed CMI (low CD4 count) The 2003 smallpox vaccination program in the US included 10 HIV-infected military personnel who were inadvertently vaccinated. All had CD4 counts > 280/mm³, all had a "take," indicating an immune response, and all tolerated the vaccine well (CID 2004;38:1320)

a Recommendations of Advisory Committee on Immunization Practices (MMWR 1993;42(RR-4); Clin Micro Rev 1998;11:1) and USPHS/IDSA committee on prevention of opportunistic infections (MMWR 2002;51(RR-6).
b Average wholesale price from: Price Alert, Databank, San Bruno, CA, June 2004.

6—Antiretroviral Therapy
Management of HIV-Infected Patients
and Post-Exposure Prophylaxis

Historical Perspective

Three nearly simultaneous developments revolutionized HIV care during 1995–1997. First, it was shown that HIV replicated at a rate that produced 10 billion virions daily throughout most of the disease (Nature 1995;373:117, 223). Second, quantitative plasma HIV RNA was introduced as a method to determine prognosis and response to therapy. The third development was the introduction of new and more potent antiretroviral agents, PIs, and NNRTIs. HAART was popularized in 1996, and by 1997, there was a 60–80% decrease in hospitalizations, deaths and AIDS-defining diagnoses. These benefits changed the image and clinical features of HIV infection and they were sustained (NEJM 1998;338:853; Ann Intern Med 2003;138:620; JAIDS 2001; 28:73; JAIDS 2003;33:321; Lancet 2003;362:1267). However, enthusiasm was tempered by some tough issues with the new therapy: 1) There was still no cure; 2) no studies clearly defined when treatment should start; 3) there was substantial evidence that HAART was associated with severe consequences, especially lipodystrophy and mitochondrial toxicity; 4) clinical experience showed convincingly that adherence was critical to achieve virologic success—in fact, the threshold for virologic failure in >50% was consumption of 70–95% of prescribed pills; and 5) there was increasing concern about resistance to antivirals both in treated patients and in newly infected patients. The result is a revision in the philosophy of care (Fig. 2) that 1) is more conservative in the recommendations for initiation of treatment, 2) is still very aggressive once the decision has been made to start HAART, 3) strongly emphasizes adherence and regimen simplification, and 4) pays substantial attention to side effects.

Current Recommendations

The following recommendations are from the Panel on Use of Antiretroviral Agents in Adults and Adolescents DHHS (www.aidsinfo.nih.gov) and the International AIDS Society—USA (JAMA 2002;288:222). Note that recommendations for antiretroviral agents change rapidly, and the most recent DHHS version is available from the HIV/AIDS Treatment Information Service website (www.aidsinfo.nih.gov.org). The tables presented here are from the June 2004 version with material from *2004 Medical Management of HIV Infection,* www.hopkins-aids.edu. Chapter 6 is organized as follows:

Antiretroviral therapy for HIV-infected patients

When to start (Tables 18–20)

What to start (Tables 21–23)

When to change therapy

Antiretroviral therapy for HIV-infected pregnant women (Tables 24–25)

Management of occupational exposure (Tables 26–28)

Table 18. Indications for Initiation of Antiretroviral Therapy
DHHS Recommendations

Clinical Category	CD4+ T Cell Count and HIV RNA	Recommendation
Acute HIV syndrome or ≤6 mo of seroconversion	Any value	Treatment may be offered, preferably in a clinical trial*
Symptomatic (AIDS, severe symptoms)	Any value	Treat*
Asymptomatic	CD4 <200 VL—any value	Treat*
Asymptomatic	CD4 200–350/mm^3 VL—(see comment)	Treatment may be offered, especially if VL >20,000 c/mL*
Asymptomatic	CD4 >350/mm^3	Defer; some experts would treat if VL >55,000 c/mL*

* Treatment assumes patient readiness

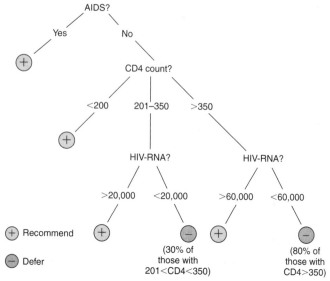

Figure 2. Treatment based on additional analysis of MACS data (Ann Intern Med 1997;126:946). Recommendation to initiate antiretrovirals in patients is defined by a 15% risk of an AIDS-defining diagnosis within 3 yr if untreated (courtesy of A. Munoz). This treatment recommendation guideline advocates antiretrovirals in patients with a 15% probability of an AIDS-defining complication in 3 years (see Table 20), and it is consistent with the DHHS guidelines.

Table 19. Initial Treatment
IAS-USA Recommendations (JAMA 2002;283:222)

- Acute HIV syndrome
- Symptomatic chronic HIV infection
- CD4 count <200/mm³
- CD4 count >200/mm³: individualize decision based on CD4 count (some authorities use a threshold of 350/mm³) rate of CD4 decline (>100/mm³/yr), viral load (>50,000–100,000 c/mL) and treatment-associated risks (toxicity and drug interactions)

Table 20. Risk of Progression to AIDS-defining Illness (1987 Definition) Based on Baseline CD4 Cell Count and Viral Load[a]

CD4 <350 + VL (copies/mL)	n	% with AIDS-defining complication[b]		
		3 yr	6 yr	9 yr
1501–7000	30	0	18.8	30.6
7001–20,000	51	8.0	42.2	65.6
20,001–55,000	73	40.1	72.9	86.2
>55,000	174	72.9	92.7	95.6
CD4 351–500 + VL (copies/mL)				
1501–7000	47	4.4	22.1	46.9
7001–20,000	105	5.9	39.8	60.7
20,001–55,000	121	15.1	57.2	78.6
>55,000	121	47.9	77.7	94.4
CD4 >500 + VL (copies/mL)				
≤1500	110	1.0	5.0	10.7
1501–7000	180	2.3	14.9	33.2
7001–20,000	237	7.2	25.9	50.3
20,001–55,000	202	14.6	47.7	70.6
>55,000	141	32.6	66.8	76.3

[a] Data from Multi-Center AIDS Cohort Study (MACS) (Ann Intern Med 1997;126:946).
[b] AIDS was defined according to 1987 CDC definition and does not include asymptomatic individuals with CD4 counts <200/mm^3.

What to Start with

Table 21. Recommendations for Initial Antiretroviral Regimen from DHHS Guidelines August 2004 (www.aidsinfo.nih.gov//guidelines)

Preferred (considered equally effective)

• Efavirenz + lamivudine* + (zidovudine, tenofovir, or stavudine**)
• Lopinavir/ritonavir + lamivudine* + (zidovudine or stavudine)

Alternatives (may be preferred in some patients)

• Efavirenz + lamivudine* + (abacavir or didanosine)
• Nevirapine + (lamivudine or emtricitabine) + (zidovudine, stavudine,** didanosine, or abacavir)
• Atazanavir + (lamivudine or emtricitabine) + (zidovudine, stavudine,** or abacavir)
• Indinavir/ritonavir + (lamivudine or emtricitabine) + (zidovudine, stavudine,** or abacavir)
• Fosamprenavir/ritonavir + (lamivudine or emtricitabine) + (zidovudine, stavudine,** or abacavir)
• Nelfinavir + (lamivudine or emtricitabine + zidovudine, stavudine,** or abacavir)
• Saquinavir (Invirase or Fortovase) + (lamivudine or emtricitabine) + (zidovudine, abacavir, or stavudine**)

---

* Lamivudine—emtricitabine appears equivalent but experience is less extensive.
** Note risk of long-term toxicity of d4T.

Table 22a. Relative Merits of Initial Regimens

Regimens	Advantages	Disadvantages
Non-nucleoside RT inhibitor-based HAART*		
EFV + 2 NRTIs	Potency Durable—4 yr data One cap/day (EFV) Minimal food effect	Neurotoxicity and rash Teratogenic—avoid in first trimester Single mutation confers class resistance
NVP + 2 NRTIs	Potency Two caps/day (NVP) No food effect Few drug interactions	Serious ADRs—hepatotoxicity and rash Contraindicated for initial Rx in women with CD4 > 250 Single mutation confers class resistance
DLV + 2 NRTIs	Increases PI levels	Minimal efficacy data Dosing—tid Single mutation confers class resistance
Protease inhibitor-based HAART**		
LPV/r + 2 NRTIs	Coformulated Potency Durable—4 yr data No PI resistance with initial failure	Nausea, diarrhea Food requirement Limited experience in pregnancy High pill burden
ATV or ATV/r + 2 NRTIs	Potency Low pill burden Once daily dosing No significant lipid effect Good GI tolerance Unique resistance mutation (50 L)	Limited experience Food requirement Hyperbilirubinemia with jaundice Absorption is acid pH-dependent
FPV/r + 2 NRTIs	Potency No food effect Favorable resistance profile Reduced lipid effect Reduced pill burden	Limited experience Rash and nausea Cross-resistance with LPV (50 V)

Table 22a. (continued)

Regimens	Advantages	Disadvantages
NFV + 2 NRTIs	Well-tolerated Extensive experience Favorable pharmacology and tolerance in pregnancy No PI cross-resistance with major mutation (30 N)	Reduced potency vs other regimens Food requirement PI cross-resistance with 90 M Poor boosting with RTV Diarrhea
IDV/r + 2 NRTIs	Experience extensive	Food restriction Fluid requirement Nephrolithiasis sica-syndrome RTV combinations • 400/400 poor tolerance • 800/200 renal stones PI cross-resistance
SQV/r + 2 NRTIs	Extensive experience Extensive experience and favorable pharmacokinetics in pregnancy	High pill burden GI intolerance—less with invirase PI cross-resistance
APV or APV/r RTV		FPV preferred Poor tolerance
Triple nucleoside regimens		
AZT/3TC/ABC	Extensive experience 1 pill bid Preserves PI and NNRTI options Co-formulated	Reduced potency compared to EFV ABC hypersensitivity AZT intolerance
SQV/r + 2 NRTIs	Extensive experience Extensive experience and tolerance in pregnancy	High pill burden GI intolerance—less with invirase PI cross-resistance
APV or APV/r RTV		FPV preferred Poor GI tolerance

* All NNRTIs have the risk of class resistance with a single mutation.
** All PIs except NFV have improved pharmacology with an increased barrier to resistance when boosted with RTV; all PIs have the risk of hyperlipid-emia (except ATV) insulin resistance and fat redistribution.

Table 22b. Nucleoside Pairings

Pairing	Advantage	Disadvantage
AZT/3TC*	Extensive experience Low pill burden Co-formulated No food effect 184 V mutation slows AZT resistance	AZT toxicity risk Failure associated TAMS and cross-resistance Mitochondrial toxicity (AZT)
ABC/3TC*	Well-tolerated Avoids TAMS Co-formulated No food effect Low pill burden Potential for qd dosing	ABC hypersensitivity risk
TDF/3TC*	Well-tolerated Low pill burden Avoids TAMS Both active vs HBV Low potential for mitochondrial toxicity Once-daily regimen	Risk of cross-resistance to ABC and ddl
TDF/FTC	As above but also co-formulated	As above
AZT/ddl	Extensive experience Low pill burden	Side effects of both Risk of TAMS Complex dosing—ddl need empty stomach and AZT tolerance improved with food Mitochondrial toxicity
ddl/d4T	Extensive experience Low pill burden Once daily dosing	Toxicity—high rates of lactic acidosis, neuropathy, pancreatitis, and lipoatrophy Food effect Contraindicated in pregnancy
ddl/3TC*	Once daily Low pill burden Avoids TAMS	Minimal data ddl toxicity risk Food effect (ddl)
d4T/3TC*	Well-tolerated—short-term No food effect Low pill burden 184 V mutation slows d4T resistance	d4T toxicity risk Risk of TAMS with failure

* FTC is probably equivalent to 3TC and has potential advantage of qd dosing but less extensive experience.

Table 23. Regimens for Special Situations

Issue	Recommendation
Pregnancy potential	Avoid efavirenz
Pregnancy	Avoid efavirenz, especially in first trimester Most experience and best-tolerated are nelfinavir and saquinavir/ritonavir-based HAART TDF—use with caution due to limited experience and concern for fetal bone effect

Tuberculosis
  Latent
  Active
	Standard INH prophylaxis
	If on HAART—continue and adjust dose of PI or NNRTI for rifamycin
	Not on HAART—CD4 count < 200: delay HAART 2–8 wk; CD4 count > 200: delay HAART until TB treated

CD4 > 250 in women	Avoid nevirapine as initial treatment
Hepatic disease	Some avoid nevirapine and ritonavir Use efavirenz and all PIs with caution; dose adjustment guidance for FPV, ATV, and IDV (see Table 33) NRTIs—standard doses
Cardiovascular disease	May prefer NNRTI-based HAART or ofazanavir ± ritonavir
Methadone	May prefer HAART to avoid NNRTI-based ddI—may need dose increase
Renal failure	May want to avoid IDV and TDF because they are nephrotoxic Dose adjust all NRTIs PIs and NNRTIs—usual doses
Acute HIV Infection	An analysis of 31 reports and 4 randomized clinical trials published prior to 2004 showed no clear evidence that antiretroviral therapy introduced prior to sero-conversion has clinical benefit (AIDS 2004;18:709)

A. MANAGEMENT OF HIV-INFECTED PATIENTS
When to Start Antiretroviral Therapy
Issues in initial therapy

Adherence: There is a consistently demonstrated strong association between adherence and virologic response with good evidence that >95% of prescribed doses must be taken to get a 80% probability of achieving the therapeutic goal of "no detectable virus" with a viral load of <50 c/mL (Ann Intern Med 2000; 133:21; AIDS 2001;15:2109; Clin Infect Dis 2001;33:386/ AIDS 2000;14:357; Clin Infect Dis 2002;34:115; J Gen Intern Med 2002; 17:377). There is a somewhat paradoxical association between adherence and resistance. The highest probability of resistance is with good adherence and virologic failure. Resistance rates are highest with consumption of 70–95% of prescribed doses; with <60% of prescribed doses the rate failure is 80%, but the frequency of resistance is nil (AIDS 2003;17:1925; Clin Infect Dis 2003;37:112).

Issues to address relevant to adherence

- Be aware that the best likelihood of success is with the first two regimens; after that there is a progressive decline in probability of virologic control and a progressive decrease in therapeutic options. The patient needs to know this.
- Make sure the patient is properly informed and "ready"
- Address common problems—warn of common and important adverse reactions, food requirements, and dosing frequency.
- Address drug interaction
- Use common aids tailored to patient idiosyncracies—pill boxes, pictures, alarms, pagers, etc.
- Use facilitators—pharmacists, counselors, peers, partners, relatives, etc.
- Test knowledge with pills or pictures.
- Documentation methods—pharmacy records, questionnaires, partner, household member, pill count, blood levels, or therapeutic drug monitoring.

Monitoring virologic response

The expected response is a 1-log 10 copies/mL decrease within 1–2 wk (JAIDS 2002;30:167; Lancet 2001;358:1760), a decrease to

<500 copies/mL by 8–16 wk (JAIDS 2000;24:433; JAIDS 2000; 25:36), and a viral load <50 copies/mL by 16–24 wk.

Causes of virologic failure

- Resistance
- Failure of drug to reach target due to poor adherence, pharmacokinetics (due to malabsorption or metabolism), or drug interactions

Durability

- Durable suppression is demonstrated for 4 years with LPV/r-based HAART (AIDS 2004;18:775) and EFV-based HAART (8th CROI, Chicago, 2001, Abstract # 325).
- Resistance mutations generally evolve with a frequency that is directly correlated with the viral load and duration of treatment to the agents in the regimen, eg, the probability of resistance is increased 100-fold for a defined period if the viral load is 60,000 copies/mL compared to 600 copies/mL. Studies of HIV clones with VL < 150 copies/mL show essentially no evolution of resistance mutations over 1 year (J Infect Dis 2004;189:1452).

Expertise

Multiple studies show superior outcomes when HIV care is proved by providers with experience in this case.

- Improved survival: NEJM 1996;334:701; AIDS 1998;12:417; J Gen Intern Med 2003;18:95.
- Access to HAART:AIDS 2003;17 Suppl 3:S 79; JAIDS 2000; 24:106; J Gen Intern Med 2003;8:233
- Patient adherence to HAART: Antivir Ther 2003;8:471

The definition of expertise has generally been based on panel size with thresholds of 20–50 active patients with HIV, and this is combined with a CME expectation of 6–50 HIV-specific CME hours/year.

When to Change Therapy

The goal of antiretroviral therapy is to reduce the level of HIV RNA to as low a level as possible for as long as possible, preferably using antiretroviral regimens that preserve future options, are relatively free of side effects, and are tailored to individual patient needs for adherence.

Analysis of virologic results from many studies indicates that the post-treatment viral burden nadir is the best predictor of the durability of a sustained viral response (Lancet 2003;362:679; (www.art.cohort-collaboration.org). Optimal results are achieved with undetectable virus using an assay with a threshold of 20–50 copies/mL. Studies also show that <5% of all AIDS-defining complications occur in patients with a viral burden of <5000 copies/mL, suggesting that thresholds that define virologic failure and clinical failure may be different. However, virologic failure leads to resistance, which in theory will eventually lead to clinical failure. Viral load levels <50 copies/mL suggest persistent low-level viremia, but this does not appear to be associated with the evolution of resistance mutations (J Infect Dis 2004;189:1452). The frequency of resistance mutations with higher viral loads depends on the level and duration of viremia, and the antiviral pressure exerted.

The probability of achieving the goal of <50 copies/mL can be crudely predicted by the decay slope in plasma HIV RNA levels, which should show a decrease of 0.75–1.0 $\log_{10}$ copies/mL at 1 wk (Lancet 2001;358:1760; J AIDS 2002;30:167); a VL <5000 copies/mL at 4 wk, <500 copies/mL by 8–16 wk and <50 copies/mL at 16–24 wk (Ann Intern Med 2001;135:954; JAIDS 2000;24:433). It should be emphasized that the ability to achieve these goals at the designated time is highly contingent on the baseline viral load. Once the goal of therapy has been achieved, therapy should be continued indefinitely with monitoring of HIV RNA levels at 3- to 4-mo intervals and CD4 counts at 3- to 6-mo intervals.

A major goal of antiretroviral therapy is viral suppression as indicated by HIV RNA levels. Changes in therapy based on inadequate virologic response should be confirmed using at least two viral load measurements at a time of clinical stability, bearing in mind that the 95% confidence interval for the test is about 3-fold. The CD4 count often increases 30–50/mm^3 in the first 3–4 mo, largely due to redistribution. With virologic suppression the subsequent rate of increase averages 100–200/mm^3/yr (JID 2002;185:471; AIDS 2001;15:983; CID 2001;32:1231). Discordant changes occur in up to 20% of patients (JID

2001;183:1328). In most cases, therapeutic decisions are based on viral load responses rather than CD4 counts, although the CD4 count is probably a better indicator of susceptibility to an AIDS-deficiency complication.

How to Change Therapy

Intolerance: Single drug substitutions are appropriate if virologic goals have been achieved. These are usually within class unless it is a class-associated ADR.

First regimen failure: The probability of achieving virologic control is good. It is important to determine the reason for failure, by review of relevant history (adherence, food issues, drug interactions, etc) and resistance testing. The latter provides guidance for drug selection in the next regimen. The three issues to address are for a regimen that is: (1) realistic for the patient; (2) likely to achieve virologic control; and (3) preserve future options. The latter is particularly important in early stage disease. As expected, extensive experience shows that the best results are achieved with a new regimen using a new class such as NNRTI-based HAART after virologic failure with PI-based HAART in a NNRTI treatment-naive patient (CID 2004; 38: 1613).

Treatment failure: There are three definitions from the 2004 DHHS guidelines

1. *Virologic failure* as previously defined. The viral load levels that define virologic failure are: VL >400 copies/mL at 24 wk, VL >50 copies/mL at 48 wk or a confirmed viral rebound to >400 copies/mL after viral suppression. These observations should prompt careful scrutiny of the reason, with adherence and resistance being the major concerns. This is the form of failure that is most important to address and it should be done in a timely fashion.
2. *Immunologic failure* is defined as the failure of the CD4 count to increase by 25–50/mm^3 in 1 year. The average increase is 100–150/mm^3. The disconnect sometimes observed between viral suppression and CD4 rebound is not understood. There does not appear to be an analysis or intervention that can be recommended. Some have suggested IL-2, but without adequate data to make this a recommendation.

3. *Clinical failure* is defined as a new AIDS-defining opportunistic infection or relapse of a prior OI after at least three months of otherwise successful antiretroviral therapy. Caution is necessary to exclude immune reconstitution syndromes in this definition. There is no clear explanation or antiretroviral intervention to deal with this.

Multiple regimen failure: The probability of virologic control becomes increasingly difficult with multiple failures. In such cases, the goals of therapy may change to preserving the CD4 count and preventing opportunistic infections. Some of the strategies for patients with multiple failures are

- Use of enfuvirtide (T-20)—an agent that has proven effective in patients with 3-class resistance (NEJM 2003;348:2175; NEJM 2003;348:2186). Enfuvirtide requires administration by subcutaneous injections bid; there are local hypersensitivity reactions that require rotation of injection sites, and this drug cannot be advocated unless there is at least one additional active antiretroviral agent to pair it with. Despite these limitations, the virologic responses achieved have been impressive.
- Experimental agents that target multiresistant strains of HIV may be an option through an expanded access program or by referral to a trial.
- Combinations of PIs or PIs plus NNRTIs may be an option according to guidance in dosing (Table 22a) and resistance testing.
- MegaHAART: This refers to the use of 6–7 antiretroviral agents including "re-cycling." The experience in reducing viral load is variable and the toxicity rates are high (JAIDS 2002;29:58; AIDS 2004;18:217).
- Structured treatment interruption: The theory is that discontinuation of the failing regimen will eliminate antiviral pressure and allow "wild-type virus" that is sensitive to antiviral agents to return. This seems a flawed concept and has not worked in practice. The largest study (NEJM 2003;349:837) showed treatment discontinuation was associated with a median 1.2 log log 10/mL increase in viral load, a rapid decrease in CD4 cell count that averaged 80/mm^3 at 3 months and multiple AIDS-defining OIs. Nevertheless,

Katlana et al. have reported better outcomes with shorter periods of treatment interruption (8 vs 16 wk) and an aggressive MegaHAART regimen when treatment was resumed (AIDS 2004; 18:217).

- Continuation of a failed regimen: When treatment options are limited or nil, it is recommended that the failing regimen be continued because discontinuation is associated with the changes noted—a rapid increase in viral load and decrease in CD4 count. It is unclear if this result is due to reduced fitness of the viral strains with resistance mutations or partial activity of the antiretroviral regimen.

Blips.   Blips are transient elevations in viral load usually to 50–500 copies/mL. They are seen in 40–50% of patients who achieve levels of <50 copies/mL. They appear to be meaningless and probably reflect the imprecision of viral load testing. Nevertheless, it is important to show they are inconsistent.

Intensification.   Intensification is addition of a drug to intensify a virologic response that is good but not as profound as desired. This may be early in the viral decay curve (4–12 wks) or could occur with confirmed slight elevations after virologic success. Common intensification efforts are the addition of TDF or ABC to dual nucleosides or the addition of RTV to regimens with a single PI other than NFV. Intensification by adding a third class drug is generally not recommended.

Fitness.   The concept is that multiply mutated HIV strains may have reduced replicative capacity. The implication is that antiretroviral agents in the face of multiple resistance mutations and virologic failure may achieve clinical benefit despite the bad numbers. Evidence to support the concept is the rapid decline in CD4 count that accompanies return of wild-type HIV when failed therapy is stopped (NEJM 2001;344:472). Some companies now provide "fitness assays," but the value and indications for such tests have not been tested.

Viral Load and CD4 Disconnect.   The failure of the expected inverse correlation of the viral load and CD4 count appears to apply in up to 35% of patients and is largely unexplained (Ann Intern Med 2000;133:401; JID 2000;181:946).

Treatment success: Pulse therapy.

Patients with immune recovery may safely discontinue therapy for periods dictated by the ensuing decline in CD4 count and the threshold for restarting. The experience is largely anecdotal but consistently successful (J Infect Dis 2002;186:851; Clin Infect Dis 2003;37:1541; AIDS 2003;17:F33). There is one prospective study that is also supportive (AIDS 2004;18:439). The usual criteria are viral control with a CD4 rebound to >500/mm^3 and suspension of therapy with monitoring of the CD4 decline and viral load rebound. The indications for reinitiation of antiretroviral therapy are arbitrary but many use the CD4 threshold of 350/mm^3. The period of therapy is highly variable, but usually averages about 1 yr with great individual patient variation. The most important indicator of the anticipated time off treatment by these guidelines is the nadir CD4 count prior to antiretroviral therapy (AIDS 2004;18:439). There are three admonitions with this strategy:

1) There must be awareness that there will be a prompt and substantial decrease in CD4 count averaging 100–200/mm^3 in the first month accompanied by virologic rebound, usually to pretreatment levels. The CD4 decline is great if the pretreatment level was <200/mm^3.
2) The patient needs to be warned about the risks of transmission associated with a high viral load.
3) When discontinuing antiretroviral agents, it is appropriate to stop them all at once with the exception of NNRTIs. Both NVP and EFV have long half lives, incurring the risk of prolonged monotherapy with subtherapeutic levels and the associated theoretical risk of resistance. One potential solution is to stop these drugs 2 wk early and substitute a PI.

Short cycle intermittent therapy (SIT):   This strategy uses HAART with periodic scheduled treatment interruptions in patients who have achieved virologic control and immune improvement. The goal is to reduce cost and side effects of ART and to provide a "drug holiday" for pill-weary patients. The best-documented successful experience is with 1 wk on and 1 wk off after there has been virologic control (<500 copies/mL) for >6 mo and a CD4 count >300/mm^3 using IDV/r-based HAART. (PNAS 2001;98:15161) or EFV-based HAART (JID 2004; 189:1974). The preliminary data are supportive with retention of virologic control and no evolution of resistance at 1 yr; nevertheless, the total patients studied in both trials is only 17, and more studies are needed before this can be advocated. Somewhat paradoxically, others have reported that the greatest risk for virologic failure and resistance in retrospective reviews is repeated drug holidays (CID 2004':1311).

Management of HIV Infection in Pregnant Patients

(Recommendations of the US Public Health Service, June 23, 2004 (http://AIDSinfo.nih.gov) (see Table 78 and 79)

Untreated pregnant woman prior to labor

- Standard evaluation
- Standard criteria for antiretroviral agents but modified regimen according to risks and benefits as applied to pregnancy
- AZT prophylaxis regimen* should be started after first trimester regardless of HIV viral load
- AZT plus additional drugs should be recommended based on clinical status and CD4 count and viral load >1000
- Women in first trimester may delay initiating ART until after 10–12 wk gestation
- Women receiving ART, with VL >1000 copies/ml at 36 weeks should be offered a C-section at 38 wk

Women receiving antiretroviral therapy

- Continue ART; include AZT in the regimen after the first trimester when possible
- Women in the first trimester should be informed of the risks and benefits of ART. Therapy may be continued; if discontinued, then all drugs should be stopped and reintroduced simultaneously
- Regardless of antepartum ART, AZT is recommended for intrapartum and for the newborn*

Untreated women in labor

- Treatment options
  1) Intrapartum AZT,* then AZT × 6 wk for the newborn*
  2) Intrapartum AZT + 3TC,* then AZT + 3TC × 1 wk for the newborn.

3) Intrapartum single-dose NVP at onset of labor, then one dose at 48 hr for the newborn
4) Two-dose NVP regimen + AZT,* then AZT at 6 wk for newborn*

- Postpartum evaluation for ART

Resistance testing

- AZT monotherapy is an option if the VL is <1000 copies/mL; the risk of resistance should be explained
- Indications for resistance tests are the same as without pregnancy: acute HIV and virologic failure
- With documented or suspicion of AZT resistance, this drug should still be given the intrapartum and infant components of the ACTG 076 protocol
- If ART needs to be discontinued for any reason—stop all drugs together

*ACTG 076 protocol

Antepartum: Oral AZT (600 mg/d in 2 or 3 doses) initiated at 14–34 wk

Intrapartum: IV AZT (2 mg/kg over 1 hr, then 1 mg/kg/hr until delivery

Postpartum: Oral AZT for newborn 2 mg/kg q 6 hr × 6 wk starting at 8–12 wk

Table 24. Antiretroviral Drug Selection in Pregnancy: Recommendations of the U.S. Public Health Service Task Force for Use of Antiretroviral Drugs in Pregnant Women, Updated Version June 23, 2004

Agent	Pharmacokinetics	Concerns
Nucleosides and nucleotides		
Recommended		
• AZT	Not altered	Safe for mother and not teratogenic
• 3TC	Not altered	Well-tolerated and not teratogenic
Alternatives		
• ddI	Not altered	Case reports of fatalities with ddI and d4T lactic acidosis
• FTC	Not studied	No studies
• d4T	Not altered	Avoid ddI and d4T (see ddI)
• ABC	Not studied	Hypersensitivity rates with pregnancy unknown
Inadequate data to recommend		
• TDF	Not studied	Animal studies show decreased bone growth and bone porosity
Not recommended		
• ddC		Teratogenic potential in rodent model
Protease inhibitors		
Recommended		
• NFV	Adequate levels with 1250 mg bid	Well-tolerated, Extensive experience Concern suboptimal viral load suppression
• SQV/r (Fortovase)	Adequate levels with 800/100 bid	Well-tolerated
Alternatives		
• IDV	Undergoing study with 800/100 bid	Theoretical increase in indirect bilirubinemia in infant and lower blood levels in pregnancy
• LPV/r	Undergoing study with 400/100 bid	Limited experience
• RTV	Reduced levels in pregnancy	Limited experience
Insufficient data		
• APV/r	Not studied	Limited experience
• ATV	Not studied	Theoretical concern for increased risk of elevated indirect bilirubin No studies in people
• APV and FPV	Not studied	No studies
Non-nucleoside RT inhibitors		
Recommended		
• NVP	Not altered	Not teratogenic Risk of rash and of hepatotoxicity, especially with baseline CD4 > 250
Not recommended		
• EFV	Not studied	Teratogenic with neural tube defects with 1st trimester exposure
• DLV	Not studied	Teratogenic in rodent studies

B. PREVENTION OF PERINATAL TRANSMISSION— ACTG 076 AND BEYOND

More recent studies show that HAART reduces perinatal transmission to 1–2% (NEJM 2002;346:1879). The rate is strongly correlated with VL at the time of delivery (NEJM 1999;13:407). Cesarean section has established merit in reducing perinatal transmission if done electively (BMJ 2001;322:511). The current recommendations are:

1. HAART for any pregnant woman with a CD4 count <350/mm^3 *or* VL >1000 c/mL (Table 24)
2. Include AZT in the regimen; avoid EFV and d4T/ddI
3. Offer elective cesarean section at 38 weeks if VL >1000/mL.
4. If VL <1000 c/mL and CD4 >350/mm offer AZT monotherapy or HAART during pregnancy.

Antiretroviral Pregnancy Registry

Care providers with HIV-infected pregnant women treated with antiretroviral agents should report observations to the following:

Antiretroviral Pregnancy Registry
115 North Third Street, Suite 306
Wilmington NC 28401
Tel: 800-258-4263 or 910-251-9087
Fax: 800-800-1052

C. POST-EXPOSURE PROPHYLAXIS FOR HEALTH CARE WORKERS

Risk for Transmission

A total of 23 studies of needlesticks among health care workers demonstrate HIV transmission in 20 of 6135 (0.33%) exposed to an HIV-infected source (Ann Intern Med 1990;113:740). With mucosal surface exposure, there was one transmission in 1143 exposures (0.09%), and there were no transmissions in 2712 skin exposures.

As of June 2003, there were 57 health care workers in the United States who had occupationally acquired HIV infection as indicated by seroconversion in the context of an exposure to an HIV-infected source. There are an additional 138 health care workers who had possible occupationally acquired HIV; these latter health care workers did not have documented seroconversion in the context of an exposure. Of the 57 confirmed cases, 1) the major occupations were nurses (23), laboratory technicians (20), and physicians (6); 2) all transmissions involved blood or bloody body fluid except for three involving laboratory workers exposed to HIV viral cultures; 3) exposures were percutaneous in 46, mucocutaneous in five, and both in two; and 4) to date there are no confirmed seroconversions in surgeons and no seroconversions with exposures to a suture needle.

A retrospective care control study of 33 HCW who seroconverted compared to 739 controls showed the risks for seroconversion were related to the viral inoculum size, depth of injury, and AZT prophylaxis (MMWR 1996;45:468; NEJM 1997;337:1485). AZT prophylaxis was associated with a 79% reduction in transmission. Nevertheless, a more recent follow-up from the CDC shows 21 cases of HIV transmission to exposed HCW despite AZT prophylaxis (NEJM 2003;348:826).

PHS Recommendations for Post-exposure Prophylaxis (PEP)

Step 1. Determine exposure code (p 84)
Step 2. Determine HIV status code (p 85)
Step 3. PEP recommendations based on exposure category (EC) and HIV RNA level in the source (p 86)

Table 25. Risk of Transmission with Occupational Exposure to Blood-Borne Viruses

Agent	Prevalence		Risk (Needlestick)	Intervention
	General Population	IDU Patients		
HIV	0.3%	10–40%	0.3%	Antiretroviral agents
HCV	1.8%	70–80%	2–3%	None (early therapy)
HBV*	0.2–0.9%	5–10%	eAg + 22% eAg − 1–6%	HBIG Vaccine

* Assumes unvaccinated HCW and HBsAg-positive source.

Comments regarding recommendations follow.

- **Drug selection.** The only drug with established merit for reducing HIV transmission with needlestick injuries is AZT (Retrovir). The rationale for recommending AZT plus 3TC (lamivudine) is based on the greater antiretroviral activity of this combination when given to patients with established infection. The addition of a PI reflects greater antiviral potency with the recommendation for high-risk injuries and settings in which resistance to AZT and/or 3TC is anticipated based on the treatment regimen of the source. The preference for indinavir or nelfinavir is based on tolerance, bioavailability, and drugs available in 1997, when the guidelines were written. The issue of drug selection has become more complex owing to the availability of 20 antiretroviral agents, concerns about toxicity, and concern about resistance in the source strain. Drugs often favored now owing to tolerance and potency for combination with AZT/3TC are lopinavir (Kaletra), Invirase, atazanavir, or fosamprenavir, and for better NRTI tolerance some prefer d4T or TDF. If the source is known to have virologic failure while receiving antiretroviral drugs, the options are the standard regimen or a regimen based on established or suspected susceptibilities. NVP is to be avoided because of hepatic necrosis (MMWR 2001;49: 1153). Efavirenz and abacavir should usually be avoided because they cause serious reactions including hypersensitivity (abacavir), or cognitive problems (efavirenz); in each case the reactions are most common in the first month of treatment, which represents the entire course of treatment. There is interest in enfuvirtide (T20) for its unique action in blocking viral entry but no experience or official recommendation; this might be considered with serious exposures.
- **Side effects.** Side effects according to the PEP Registry with 492 occupational exposures managed with standard CDC recommended regimens of AZT/3TC or AZT/3TC plus IDV or NFV are: nausea—57%, fatigue—38%, headache—18%, vomiting—16%, diarrhea—14%. The number who discontinued prophylaxis because of toxicity was 54% (Infect Control Hosp Epidemiol 2000;21:780). Stavudine

(d4T) or tenofovir is an appropriate alternative for those who do not tolerate AZT, although AZT is the only drug with established efficacy. There are few side effects with 3TC. Recipients of indinavir must take >48 oz of fluid daily to reduce the probability of renal calculi. Recipients of Lopinavir and nelfinavir should be warned of diarrhea.

- **Timing.** Prophylaxis should be initiated as rapidly as possible after exposure, preferably within 1–2 hr. Animal studies show no benefit when treatment is delayed 24–36 hr (JID 1993;168:1490; NEJM 1995;332:444); nevertheless, the CDC recommends prophylaxis with an allowable delay of up to 1–2 wk with high-risk exposures. The Hopkins program includes a 72-hr "starter pack" to promote early prophylaxis when the health care worker is undecided. There is also a service to deliver initial doses to the operating room to prevent the need to break scrub.
- **Monitoring.** HIV serology is performed at baseline, 6 wk, 12 wk, and 6 mo. We are aware of three health care workers who seroconverted at >6 mo after occupational exposure. For patients who receive post-exposure prophylaxis, the drug toxicity monitoring should include a CBC and hepatic and renal function tests at baseline and 2 wk after treatment is initiated.

Management of occupational exposure (MMWR 2001;50 [RR-1])

General

Immediate care: Wash wounds and skin with alcohol; flush mucous membranes with water

Determine risk: 1. Type of fluid-blood, visibly bloody fluid, other potentially infectious fluid or tissue and concentrated virus

2. Type of exposure

Evaluate source: 1) Test source for HBsAg, anti-HCV, and anti-HIV (rapid testing for HIV preferred using SUDS or Ora-Quick, which may provide results within 20 min).

2) Unknown source—access risk for HIV, HCV, HBV

3) Do not test discarded needles, syringes etc.

Evaluate exposed HCW: HBV vaccination and vaccine response

Hepatitis C Exposure

- Source—test anti-HCV and confirm positives with quantative HCV PCR
- HCW-test anti HCV + ALT at baseline and at 3–6 mo post exposure. Confirm positive serology with quantitative HCV PCR
- HCV RNA test at 4–6 wk (optional) to detect acute HCV prior to seroconversion. Most are asymptomatic and have an elevated ALT at this stage.
- No prophylaxis recommended because many clear HCV spontaneously and the role of HCV treatment at this stage is unknown. (J Infect Dis 1996;173:822; Clin Microbiol Rev 2003;16:546).

Hepatitis B Exposure (Table 26)

- Source—test for HBVsAg
- Management depends on vaccine status of HCW

HIV Exposure (Table 27 and Table 28)

- Recommended regimens
  - *2 drug PEP:* AZT/3TC (standard) or ddI/d4T, d4T/3TC, AZT/ddI, TDF/3TC
  - *3 drug PEP:* Above plus a PI or a boosted PI. Many recommended LPV/r

Table 26. Management of HBV Exposure

Vaccine Status Health Care Worker	Features of Source	
	HBs Ag Positive	Source Unknown
Unvaccinated	HBIG* + vaccine (3 doses)	HBV vaccine (3 doses)
Vaccinated responder**	No Rx	No Rx
Nonresponder	HBIG × 1 + vaccine series or HBIG × 2***	Rx as source positive if high risk
Antibody status unknown	Test anti-HBs • >10 mIU/mL—No Rx • <10 mIU/mL—vaccine booster	

* HBIG = Hepatitis B Immune Globulin. Dose is 0.06 ml/kg IM. Give ASAP and ≤7 days.
** Responder defined by antibody level ≥10 mIU/mL.
*** HBIG + vaccine series preferred for non-responders who did not complete the 3-dose series; HBIG × 2 doses preferred if 2-vaccine series and no response.

Table 27. Percutaneous Injuries

Exposure	Status of Source		Unknown
	Low Risk	High Risk*	
Not severe (solid needle superficial)	2 drug PEP**	3 drug PEP**	Usually none; consider 2 drug PEP***
Severe (large bore, visible blood on device, needle in pt artery or vein)	3 drug PEP**	3 drug PEP**	Usually none; consider 2 drug PEP***

* Low risk: Asymptomatic HIV or VL < 1,500 c/mL; high risk: Symptomatic HIV, AIDS seroconversion, high viral load.
** Concern for drug resistance—start prophylaxis and consult expert.
*** Consider 2 drug PEP if source high risk or exposure is from unknown source where HIV likely.

> *Modify* according to anticipated or measured resistance in source strain
>
> *Drugs to avoid:* Nevirapine, efavirenz, abacavir and ddC

- Monitoring

  HIV serology repeated at 6 wk, 3 mo and 6 mo

- Counseling of health care worker

  Transmission prophylaxis: Safe sex or no sex especially during first 6–12 wk

  Pregnancy: Pregnancy should not preclude PEP, but should avoid efavirenz and combination of d4T + ddI

  Toxicity: Frequency of side effects—74%, most commonly nausea, fatigue, headache, vomiting, diarrhea (see Infect Control Hosp Epidemiol 2000;21:780)

Table 28. Mucocutaneous Exposure

Exosure	Status of source		Unknown
	Low risk**	High risk**	
Small volumes	Consider 2 drug PEP	2 drug PEP	Usually no PEP; consider 2 drug PEP***
Large volume	2 drug PEP	3 drug PEP	Usually no PEP; consider 2 drug PEP***

* Non-intact skin = dermatitis, abrasion, wound.
** Low risk—asymptomatic or VL <1,500 c/mL.
High risk: symptomatic HIV, AIDS, acute seroconversion, high viral load.
*** Consider if source has HIV risk factors or exposure from unknown source where HIV likely.

7—Antiretroviral Agents

Table 29. Antiretroviral Drugs Approved by FDA for HIV

Trade Name	Generic Name (abbreviation)	Firm	FDA Approval Date
Retrovir	zidovudine, AZT	GlaxoSmithKline	Mar 1987
Videx	didanosine, ddI	Bristol-Myers Squibb	Oct 1991
Hivid	zalcitabine, ddC	Hoffman-La Roche	Jun 1992
Zerit	stavudine, d4T	Bristol-Myers Squibb	Jun 1994
Epivir	lamivudine, 3TC	GlaxoSmithKline	Nov 1995
Invirase	saquinavir, SQV, hgc	Hoffman-La Roche	Dec 1995
Fortovase	saquinavir, SQV, sgc	Hoffman-La Roche	Nov 1997
Norvir	ritonavir, RTV	Abbott Laboratories	Mar 1996
Crixivan	indinavir, IDV	Merck	Mar 1996
Viramune	nevirapine, NVP	Boehringer Ingelheim	Jun 1996
Viracept	nelfinavir, NFV	Agouron Pharmaceuticals	Mar 1997
Rescriptor	delavirdine, DLV	Pharmacia & Upjohn	Apr 1997
Combivir	zidovudine and iamivudine	Glaxo Wellcome	Sep 1997
Sustiva	efavirenz, EFV	DuPont Pharmaceuticals	Sep 1998
Ziagen	abacavir, ABC	GlaxoSmithKline	Feb 1999
Agenerase	amprenavir, APV	GlaxoSmithKline	Apr 1999
Kaletra	lopinavir/ritonavir (LPV/r)	Abbott Laboratories	Sep 2000
Trizivir	zidovudine and lamivudine and abacavir	GlaxoSmithKline	Nov 2000
Viread	tenofovir (TDF)	Gilead	Oct 2001
Enfuvirtide	fuzeon (T20)	Roche	April 2003
Epzicom	lamivudine and abacavir	GlaxoSmithKline	July 2004
Truvada	tenofovir and emtricitabine	Gilead	July 2004

Table 30. Nucleoside Analogs

Generic name:	Zidovudine (AZT, ZDV)	Didanosine (ddI)	Zalcitabine (ddC)	Stavudine (d4T)	Lamivudine (3TC)	Abacavir (ABC)	Tenofovir (TDF)	Emtricitabine (FTC)
Trade name:	Retrovir	Videx and Videx EC	Hivid	Zerit and Zerit XR	Epivir	Ziagen	Viread	Glaxo
How supplied	100 mg caps 300 mg tabs IV vials 10 mg/mL 300 mg + 3TC 150 mg as Combivir 300 mg + 3TC 150 mg + abacavir 300 mg as Trizivir	Buffered tabs: 25, 50, 100, 150, and 200 mg Videx EC: 125, 200, 250, and 400 mg caps	0.375 and 0.75 mg tabs	15, 20, 30, and 40 mg caps 1 mg/mL oral sdn Zerit XR 100, 75 mg caps	150, 300 mg tabs 10 mg/mL oral soln 150 mg with AZT 300 mg as Combivir 300 mg + ABC 300 mg as Trizivir 300 mg + ABC 600 mg as epzicom	300 mg tabs 20 mg/mL oral soln 300 mg + 3TC 150 mg + AZT as Trizivir 600 mg + 3TC 300 mg as epzicom	300 mg tab 300 mg + FTC 200 mg as Truvada	200 mg caps 200 mg + TDF 300 mg as Truvada
Dosing recommendations	300 mg bid Combivir 1 tab bid Trizivir 1 tab bid	<60 kg Videx EC 250 mg qd Videx tabs 250 mg qd or 125 mg bid >60 kg Videx EC 400 mg qd Videx tabs 400 mg qd or 200 mg bid With TDF: 250 mg qd	0.75 mg tid	>60 kg: 40 mg bid or XR 100 mg qd <60 kg: 30 mg bid or XR75 mg qd	150 mg bid Combivir tab bid or 300 mg qd Trizivir: 1 tab bid Epzicom 1 qd	300 mg bid Trizivir 1 tab bid Epzicom 1 qd	300 mg qd Truvada 1 qd	200 mg qd Truvada 1 qd
Oral bio-availability	60%	30%–40%	85%	86%	86%	83%	25-39%	90%

Food effect	None, but better tolerated with food	Levels ↓55% Buffered: Take >1 hr before or >2 hr after meal Videx EC: Take >2 hr before or >2 hr after meal	None	None	None	None Alcohol ↑ABC levels 41%	Levels ↑ Take with meal	No effect
Serum half-life	1.1 hr	1.6 hr	1.2 hr	1.0 hr	3–6 hr	1.5 hr	17 hr	10 hr
Intracellular T½	3 hr	25–40 hr	3 hr	3.5 hr	12 hr	12 hr	10–50 hr	?
CNS penetration (% serum levels)	60%	20%	20%	30–40%	10%	30%	?	?
Elimination	Metabolized to Glucuronide (GAZT) Renal excretion of GAZT	Renal excretion—50%	Renal excretion—70%	Renal excretion—50%	Renal excretion—unchanged	Metabolized Renal excretion of metabolites—82%	Renal excretion	Renal excretion
Major toxicity Class toxicity*	Bone marrow suppression; anemia, and/or neutropenia Subjective: GI intolerance headache, insomnia, asthenia	Pancreatitis Peripheral neuropathy GI intolerance nausea, diarrhea Videx EC has fewer GI side effects	Peripheral neuropathy Stomatitis	Peripheral neuropathy Pancreatitis Lipoatrophy Hyper-lipidemia Ascending paralysis	Minimal toxicity	Hyper-sensitivity (5%), with fever, nausea, vomiting, malaise, morbilliform rash**	Occasional GI intolerance Fanconi syndrome—esp with renal insufficiency	Minimal toxicity
Clinical monitoring	CBC q 3 mo	Peripheral neuropathy	Peripheral neuropathy	Peripheral neuropathy	Peripheral neuropathy	—	—	—

* Class toxicity: Lactic acidosis with hepatic steatosis is a potentially life-threatening toxicity with use of this class. Frequency: d4T/ddI > d4T > ddI > AZT = 3TC = FTC = ABC > TDF

** Hypersensitivity reactions to abacavir may be life threatening (see p 118).

Table 31. Non-Nucleoside Reverse Transcriptase Inhibitors

Generic name:	Nevirapine	Delavirdine	Efavirenz
Trade name:	Viramune	Rescriptor	Sustiva
Form	200 mg tabs: 50 mg/5 mL oral susp	100, 200 mg tabs	50, 100, 200 mg caps 600 mg tab
Dosing recommendations	200 mg PO qd × 14 days, then 200 mg PO bid	400 mg PO tid	600 mg PO qd at hs
Oral bioavailability	>90%	85%	42%
Food effect	No effect Take without regard to meals	No effect Take without regard to meals	Increased 50% with high fat meal Take on empty stomach
Serum half-life	25–30 hr	5.8 hr	40–55 hr
Elimination	Metabolized by cytochrome P-450 (3A4 inducer): 80% excreted in urine (glucuronidated metabolites, <5% unchanged), 10% in feces	Metabolized by cytochrome P-450 (3A4 inhibitor): 51% excreted in urine (<5% unchanged), 44% in feces	Metabolized by cytochrome P-450 enzymes (3A4 mixed inhibitor/inducer); 14–34% excreted in urine, 16–61% in feces

Drug interactions	Induces cytochrome P-450 3A4 enzymes Contraindicated drugs: None PI interactions (see Table 36, p 99) Nevirapine reduces ketoconazole levels 63% (not recommended); decreases methadone levels significantly; titrate methadone dose Drugs that reduce nevirapine levels: Rifampin 37% (not recommended), rifabutin 16% (use standard dose NVP) Fewest drug interactions of this class	Inhibits cytochrome P-450 3A4 enzymes Contraindicated drugs: Terfenadine, astemizole, ergot derivatives, triazolam, midazolam, cisapride, rifabutin, rifampin, H₂ blockers, proton pump inhibitors, simvastatin, lovastatin Delavirdine increases levels of clarithromycin, dapsone, quinidine, warfarin, sildenafil Antacids and buffered ddI: Separate administration by >1 hr PI interactions (see Table 36, p 99)	Inhibits and induces cytochrome P-450 3A4 enzymes Contraindicated drugs: Astemizole, midazolam, triazolam, cisapride, ergot alkaloids, terfenadine Rifampin—EFV ↓ 25% use 800 mg/d. Rifabutin—RBT ↓ 35%; use RBT 450—600 mg 3 ×/wk PI interactions (see Table 36, p 99) Methadone: May decrease levels of methadone—monitor
Major toxicity Class toxicity*	Symptomatic hepatitis often with rash and fever ± hepatic necrosis; this may be fatal even if NVP is discontinued Risk is 11% in women with CD4 count >250 and 2% with lower CD4 counts Most cases occur in first 6–18 wk of treatment Rash (15–30%) requires discontinuation in 7%; rare cases of Stevens-Johnson syndrome	Rash (10–15%); headaches Hepatic toxicity	Dizziness, "disconnectedness," somnolence, insomnia, bad dreams, confusion, amnesia, agitation, hallucinations, poor concentration—40%, usually resolves after 2–3 wk; take hs *Rash (5–10%)—requires discontinuation in 1–7%; rare reports of Stevens-Johnson syndrome Teratogenic in cynomolgus monkeys and ≥3 reported cases of neural tube defects when given in first trimester to women. Avoid in pregnancy and with pregnancy potential
Clinical monitoring	Liver function tests baseline, wk 2 and 4, then q mo × 3 mo, then q 3 mo	None	None

* Class toxicity: Rash that may be severe; mechanism is not established; most common and severe with nevirapine.

Table 32. Protease Inhibitors

Generic name:	Indinavir	Ritonavir	Saquinavir		Nelfinavir	Amprenavir	Lopinavir/ ritonavir	Atazanavir	Fosamprenavir
Trade name:	Crixivan	Norvir	Invirase	Fortovase	Viracept	Agenerase	Kaletra	Reyataz	Lexiva
Form	200, 333, 400 mg caps	100 mg caps 600 mg/7.5 mL oral solution	200 mg caps (hard gel); 500 mg tabs (avail 1/05)	200 mg caps (soft gel)	250, 625 mg tablets 50 mg/g oral powder	50, 150 mg caps 15 mg/mL oral solution	133 mg LPV + 33 mg RTV caps 80 mg LPV + 20 mg RTV/mL oral solution	100, 150, 200 mg caps	700 mg tabs
Usual dose	800 mg q 8h Separate buffered ddI dose by 1 hr	600 mg bid Separate buffered ddI dose by 2 hr	400 mg bid with ritonavir	1200 mg tid	750 mg tid or 1250 mg bid	1200 mg bid 1400 mg bid (oral solution)	400/100 mg (3 caps or 5 mL) bid 800/200 mg (6 caps or 10 mL) qd for ARV-naive patients only	400 mg qd; with TDF use ATV/r 300/100 qd with EFV and TDF	1400 mg bid
Boosted with RTV*	800/100 bid 400/400 bid	—	400/100 bid 1000/100 bid 1600/100 qd 2000/100 qd	400/400 bid 1000/100 bid 1600/100 qd	—	600/100 bid 1200/200 qd	—	300/100 qd	700/100 bid 1400/200 qd
Food effect	Levels decrease 77%; take 1 hr before or 2 hr after meals or with low-fat snack or skim milk No food effect with IDV/RTV	Levels increased 15%; take with food if possible to improve tolerability	No food effect when taken with RTV	Levels increase 6×; take with large meal No food effect with RTV	Levels increase 2-3×; take with meal or snack, preferably high-fat meal	High-fat meal reduces AUC 20%; take with or without food but avoid high-fat meal	Fat increases AUC 50-80%; take with food	Food increases AUC 70%	No Effect
Bioavailability	65% (empty stomach)	Not known	Not known	Not known	20-80%	Not known, 14% lower	Not known	Not known	Not known

Storage	Room temp	Refrigerate caps if >1 mo	Room temp	Room temp or refrigerate	Room temp	Room temp	Room temp Stable × 2 mo	Room temp	Room temp
Serum half-life	1.5–2 hr	3–5 hr	1–2 hr	1–2 hr	3.5–5 hr	7–10 hr	Lopinavir 5–6 hr	7 hr	7.7 hr
CNS penetration	Moderate	Poor	Poor	Poor	Moderate	Moderate	Not known	Not known	Moderate
Elimination	Biliary metabolism; cytochrome P-450 3A4 inhibitor	Biliary metabolism; cytochrome P-450 3A4; 3A4 inhibitor	Biliary metabolism; cytochrome P-450 3A4 inhibitor	Biliary metabolism; cytochrome P-450 3A4 inhibitor	Biliary metabolism; cytochrome P-450 3A4 inhibitor	Biliary metabolism; cytochrome P-450 3A4 inhibitor	Biliary metabolism; cytochrome P-450 3A4 inhibitor	Biliary metabolism; cytochrome P-450 3A4 inhibitor	Biliary metabolism; cytochrome P-450 3A4 inhibitor
Side effects Class reactions*	GI intoler. (10–15%) Nephrolithiasis (10–20%) interstitial nephritis (1–2%) Headache; alopecia dry skin and mucous membranes paronychia; hepatitis, thrombocytopenia; blurred vision Lab: Increase indirect bilirubinemia (inconsequential) transaminases	GI intoler. (20–40%) Paresthesias—circumoral and extremities (10%); taste perversion (10%); asthenia Lab: Increase triglycerides (60%), transaminase (10–15%) CPK, and uric acid	GI intoler. (10–20%) Miscellaneous; headache; transaminase increases	GI intoler. (20–30%) Miscellaneous: headache; transaminase increases	GI intoler. Diarrhea (10–30%) Increased transaminase	GI intoler. (10–30%) Rash (20–25% usually at 1–10 wk) Stevens-Johnson syndrome (1%) Paresthesias (10–30—perioral or peripheral) Increased transaminases	GI intoler. esp diarrhea Asthenia Increased transaminases Oral soln is 42% ETOH-disulfiram reaction	GI intoler. Increased indirect bilirubin (jaundice) Prolonged QTc Increased transaminases	GI intoler. Skin rash (19%) Increased transaminases

* Fat accumulation, lipid abnormalities, and insulin resistance are associated with the use of protease inhibitors; exception is ATV, which does not cause hyperlipidemia. Fat redistribution is a cosmetic issue, and mechanism is unknown. Patients with hypertriglyceridemia or hypercholesterolemia should be evaluated for risks of cardiovascular events and pancreatitis. Possible interventions include dietary modification, lipid-lowering agents, or discontinuation of protease inhibitors.

Table 33a. Dose Modifications in Renal or Hepatic Failure: NRTI

Drug Name	Form	Renal Failure Dosing			Liver Failure Dosing
		CrCl 30–59 ml/min	CrCl 10–29 ml/min	CrCl <10 or Dialysis	
Abacavir (ABC, Ziogen)	300 mg tab; (see also: Trizivir) 20 mg/mL po soln.	Standard			Usual
Combivir (CBV)	AZT 300 mg + 3TC 150 mg (tab)	Fixed Formulation Not recommended			Usual
Didanosine (Videx; Videx EC; ddI)	25, 50, 100, 150, 200 mg tab (buffered) 100, 167, 250 mg powder (buffered) 125, 200, 250, and 400 mg (EC caps)	>60 kg 200 mg <60 kg 125 mg/d	>60 kg 125 mg/d <60 kg 100 mg/d¶	>60 kg 125 mg/d <60 kg 75 mg/d¶	Usual
Emtricitabine (Emtriva, FTC)	200 mg cap	200 mg q48hr	200 mg q72 hr	200 mg q96 hr¶	Usual
Lamivudine (Epivir; 3TC)	150, 300 mg tab (see also: Combivir & Trizivir) 10 mg/mL po soln.	150 mg qd	150 mg × 1 then 100 mg/d	150 mg × 1 then 25–30 mg qd¶	Usual
Stavudine (Zerit; d4T)	15, 20, 30, 40 mg cap; 75, 100 mg XR cap; 1 mg/mL po soln.	>60 kg-20 mg q 12 hr <60 kg-15 mg q12 hr	>60 kg-20 mg q24 hr <60 kg-20 mg 24 hr	>60kg-20 mg q24 hr <60 kg-20mg q 24 hr¶	Usual
Tenofovir (Viread, TDF)	300 mg tab	300 mg q 2 days	300 mg 2 days/wk	300 mg q 7 days	Usual
Trizivir (TZV)	AZT 300 mg + 3TC 150 mg + ABC 300 mg(tab) 1 qd	Fixed formulation not recommended in renal or hepatic failure			Usual
Truvada		1 q 48 h	Not recommended		Usual
Zalcitabine (Hivid; ddC)	0.375, 0.75 mg tab	Standard	0.75 mg bid	.75 mg qd	Usual
Zidovudine (Retrovir, AZT)	100 cap, 300 mg tab; (see also: Combivir & Trizivir) 10 mg/mL IV soln. 10 mg/mL po soln.	300 mg bid	300 mg qd	300 mg qd	200 mg bid

¶ Give after dialysis

Table 33b. Dose Modification in Renal and Hepatic Failure: Protease Inhibitors

Drug Name	Form	Renal Failure Dosing			Liver Failure Dosing
		CrCl 30–59 ml/min	CrCl 10–29 ml/min	CrCl <10 or Dialysis	
Amprenavir (APV, Agenerase)	50, 150 mg caps 15 mg/mL po soln**	Standard		No data	CPS* 5–8: 450 mg bid CPS* 9–12: 300 mg bid
Atazanavir (Reyataz, ATV)	100, 150, and 200 mg capsules	Standard			CPS* 7–9: 300 mg qd CPS* >9: Avoid
Fosamprenavir (FPV, Lexiva)	700 mg tabs	Standard			CPS* 5–8: 700 mg bid CPS* >9: Avoid
Indinavir (IDV, Crixivan)	200, 333, 400 mg caps	Standard			600 mg q8hr
Lopinavir/Ritonavir (LPV/r) (Kaletra)	LPV 133.3 mg + RTV 33.3 mg (cap); LPV 80 mg + RTV 20 mg/mL po soln	Standard			§§
Nelfinavir (NFV, Viracept)	250, 625 mg tabs 50 mg/g powder	Standard			§§
Ritonavir (RTV, Norvir)	100 mg caps 600 mg/7.5 mL po soln	Standard			§§
Saquinavir (SQV) Fortovase (FTV) Invirase (INV)	200 mg caps	Standard			§§

* Childs-Pugh score
§§ More frequent monitoring required. Drug change or dose change could be considered on a case-by-case basis noting the risk of resistance with underdosing

Table 33c. Dose Modification in Renal and Hepatic Failure: Non-Nucleoside RT Inhibitors and Fusion Inhibitor

Non-Nucleoside Reverse Transcriptase Inhibitors (NNRTIs)

Delavirdine (DLV, Rescriptor)	100, 200 mg tabs	No effect	Standard	§§
Efavirenz (EFV, Sustiva)	50, 100, 200 mg caps, 600 mg tabs	Avoid high-fat meal	Standard	§§
Nevirapine (NVP, Viramune)	200 mg tabs 50 mg/5 mL po susp.	No effect	Standard	Standard; give after dialysis	Avoid

Fusion Inhibitors

Enfuvirtide (ENF, Fuzeon, T-20)	108 mg single-use vials to be reconstituted with 1.1 mL H20	N/A	Standard	Standard	Usual dose

§§ More frequent monitoring required. Drug change or dose change could be considered on a case-by-case basis noting the risk of resistance with underdosing

Table 34a. Drug Interactions: Nucleosides

Drug	AZT	d4T	ddl	TDF
Methadone	AZT AUC ↑40%; no dose change	d4T ↓27%; no dose change	ddl ↓41% consider ↑ddl dose or use ddl EC	No data
ddl	—	—	—	ddl ↑44% consider ddl dose reduction
Ribavirin	Inhibits AZT activation; avoid if possible	Magnifies toxicity Use with caution	Magnifies ddl toxicity; avoid	No data
ATV	—	—	Buffered ddl—take ATV 2 hr before or 1 hr after ddl; ddl EC—seperate dosing due to food restrictions	Avoid concomitant use unless ATV combined with RTV

Table 34b. Drug Interactions: Contraindicated Combinations

Class	Contraindicated Agent	ART Agents	Alternatives
Ca++ channel blocker	Bepridil	RTV, APV, ATV	—
Antiarrhythmics	Flecainide, Propafenone	RTV, LPV/r, FPV	—
	Amiodarone, quinidine	RTV	
Lipid lowering	Simvastatin, Lovastatin	All PIs, DLV	Pravastatin or Fluvastatin, possibly Atorvastatin
	Atorvastatin	NFV, LPV	Pravastatin or Fluvastatin
Antimycobacterials	Rifampin	IDV, NFV, APV, FPV, LPV/r, SQV (unless given with RTV), DLV, & ATV	Use Rifabutin*
	Rifabutin	DLV, SQV (unless used with RTV)	Rifampin or rifabutin
	Rifapentine	All PIs, NVP, DLV, EFV	Amphotericin
Antifungal	Voriconazole	RTV EFV	Alternate azole
Antihistamine	Astemizole, Terfenadine	All PIs, DLV, EFV	Loratadine, Fexofenadine, Cetirizine, or Desloratidine
Antineoplastics	Irinotecan	ATV	—
GI	Cisapride	All PIs, DLV, EFV	—
	H2 blockers, proton pump inhibitors	DLV, ATV	
Neuroleptic	Clozapine	RTV	—
	Pimozide	All PIs	—
Psychotropic	Midazolam†, Triazolam	All PIs, DLV, EFV	Temazepam, Lorazepam, or Oxazepam
Ergot alkaloids	Alprazolam	DLV	
	Ergotamine	All PIs, DLV, EFV	—
Herbs	St. John's wort	All PIs & EFV, DLV	Alternative antidepressants

* See Table 35 for Rifabutin and antiretroviral dose adjustments
† Midazolam may be used with caution as a single dose given for a procedure.

Table 35. Drug Interactions: Combinations with PIs or NNRTIs Requiring Dose Modifications

Class	Agent	ART
Antifungal	Ketoconazole	IDV-IDV 600 mg tid RTV, LPV/r—Ketoconazole ≤200 mg/d, FPV ≤400 mg/d NVP—Not recommended NFV, ATV, APV, LPV/r; IDV is OK
	Voriconazole	
Oral contraceptives	—	Additional method of contraception recommended with: RTV, NFV, APV, EFV, LPV/r, NVP, FPV. (IDV & ATV are OK) No data—SQV. DLV ↓ ethinyl estradiol by 20%
Anticonvulsants	Phenobarbital, Phenytoin, Carbamazepine	Avoid carbamazepine + IDV and phenytoin + LPV; all other combinations of NRTIs or PIs & designated anticonvulsants should be given with caution and monitoring of anticonvulsant levels or consider valproic acid)
Methadone	—	NVP and EFV may decrease methadone substantially; monitor for withdrawal. IDV has no interaction; other PIs may decrease methadone levels and require monitoring for withdrawal. Methadone decreases buffered ddI levels - consider ddI EC (no interaction).
Antibiotics	Clarithromycin	RTV, LPV/r DLV—Decrease clarithromycin dose in renal failure EFV, ATV—Consider alternative to Clarithromycin (e.g. Azithromycin)

* These recommendations apply to regimens which do not include PIs which substantially increase rifabutin levels

Table 35. Drug Interactions: Combinations with PIs or NNRTIs Requiring Dose Modifications (Cont'd.)

Class	Agent	ART
Antimycobacterials	Rifabutin	RTV combos (any dose) 150 mg qod or 150 mg 3×/wk APV 1200 mg bid + RBT 150 mg/d or 300 mg 3×/wk FPV 1400 mg bid + RBT 150 mg/d or 300 mg 3×/wk ATV 400 mg/d + RBT 150 mg/d or 150 mg 3×/wk EFV 600 mg/d + RBT 450 mg/d or 600 mg 3×/wk* IDV 1000 mg q 8h + RBT 150 mg/d or 300 mg 3×/wk LPV/r 400/100 mg + RBT 150 mg qod NFV 1000 mg tid + RBT 150 mg/d or 300 mg 3×/wk RTV 600 mg bid + RBT 150 mg qod or 150mg 3×/wk NVP 200 mg bid + RBT 300 mg/d or 300 mg 3×/wk DLV—avoid; SQV (unboosted)—avoid
	Rifampin	All PIs & NNRTIs contraindicated except RTV, RTV + SQV, or EFV using standard doses; with EFV consider EFV daily dose of 800 mg qd. NVP - use with caution and monitor LFTs with SQV/RTV—400/400 + RIF 600 mg qd or 600 mg 3×/wk
Lipid Lowering	Lovastatin, Simvastatin Atorvastatin Pravastatin	Avoid PIs and DLV; no data for EFV and NVP. PI use with caution and monitor. No dose change—RTV, SQV, LPV/r. No data-IDV, NFV, APV, and NNRTIs
Miscellaneous	Theophylline Warfarin Sildenafil Desipramine Grapefruit juice Ribavirin Antacids, H$_2$ antagonists	RTV—Monitor theophylline levels RTV, DLV, EFV—Monitor INR closely if given with any PI or NNRTI All PIs and DLV ≤ 25 mg/48 hrs RTV—Consider desipramine dose reduction IDV ↓ SQV ↑ ddI toxicity potentiated by ribavirin-avoid use ATV - seperate dosing of buffered meds by 1-2 hr, H$_2$ antagonists by 12 hr

* These recommendations apply to regimens which do not include PIs which substantially increase rifabutin levels

Table 36. PI-PI Combinations and PI-NNRTI Combinations: Effect of Drugs on Levels (AUC)/Dose

Drug Affected	Ritonavir	Saquinavir	Nelfinavir	Amprenavir	Lopinavir	Nevirapine	Delavirdine	Efavirenz	Fosamprenavir	Atazanavir
Indinavir (IDV)	IDV 400 mg bid + RTV 400 mg bid or IDV 800 mg bid + RTV 100–200 mg bid	Insufficient data	Limited data for IDV 1200 mg bid + NFV 1250 mg bid	Standard—both drugs (Limited data)	IDV 600 mg bid LPV/r standard	IDV 1000 mg bid or tid +, NVP standard	IDV 600 mg q8 h DLV standard	IDV 1000 mg q8 hr + EFV standard or IDV 800 mg bid + RTV 200 mg bid + EFV 600 mg hs	No recommendation	Not recommended
Ritonavir (RTV)	—	SQV 1000 mg bid + RTV 100 mg bid* or SQV 400 mg bid + RTV 400 mg bid* or RTV 100 mg qd + SQV 1600 or 2000 mg qd*	RTV 400 mg bid + NFV 500–750 mg bid (Limited data)	RTV 100 mg bid + APV 600 mg bid* or APV 1200 mg qd + RTV 200 mg qd	Co-formulated	Standard (both drugs)	No data	RTV 600 mg bid (500 mg bid for intolerance) + EFV 600 mg hs	FPV 1400 mg qd + RTV 200 mg qd or FPV 700 mg bid + RTV 100 mg bid	ATV 300 mg qd + RTV 100 mg qd

Table 36. (continued)

Drug Affected	Ritonavir	Saquinavir	Nelfinavir	Amprenavir	Lopinavir	Nevirapine	Delavirdine	Efavirenz	Fosamprenavir	Atazanavir
Saquinavir (SQV)	—	—	NFV 1250 mg bid + FTV 1200 mg bid (PK data) or NFV 750 mg tid + SQV 800–1200 mg tid (clinical data)	Inadequate data	SQV 800 or 1000 mg bid + LPV/r standard**	SQV 400 mg bid + RTV 400 mg bid standard or SQV 1000 mg bid + RTV 100 mg bid + NVP standard	FTV 800 mg tid + DLV standard (monitor transaminase levels)	SQV 400 mg bid + RTV 400 mg bid + EFV 600 mg hs	SQV (hgc) 1000 mg bid + FPV 700 mg bid + RTV 100–200 mg bid	SQV 1600 mg qd + FTV 100 mg qd + ATV 300 mg qd
Nelfinavir				APV 800 mg bid + NFV 750 mg tid. (Limited data)	LPV/r 4 caps bid + NFV standard (Limited data)				Not recommended	No data
Fosamprenavir					Not recommended				—	No data
Nelfinavir (NFV)			NFV 750 mg tid. + DLV 400 mg tid (limited)	NFV 750 mg tid. + APV 800 mg tid* (limited)	LPV 4 caps bid + NFV standard (limited)	Standard (both drugs)	NFV 750 mg tid + DLV 400 mg tid (limited)	Standard (both drugs)		

Nevirapine		LVP/r 4 caps bid NVP - standard (limited data)	No data	—
Efavirenz (EFV)		EFV standard + APV 1200 mg tid or APV 1200 mg bid + RTV 200 mg bid + EFV 600 mg qd	EFV standard LPV/r 4 caps bid	Not recommended / No data	—

Adapted from DHHS guidelines (www.hivatis.com, June 2004).
* Indicates option to use Invirase or Fortovase; many authorities now prefer Invirase formulation because of better GI tolerance (FTV, Fortovase).

Class Adverse Reactions

LACTIC ACIDOSIS (J AIDS 2002;31:257)

Definition.   Elevated venous lactate level (>18 mg/dL or >2 mmol/L) plus arterial pH <7.3

Symptoms.   Insidious onset of fatigue, anorexia, wasting, abdominal pain, nausea, vomiting and dyspnea (CID 2002;34: 838). May present with fulminant hepatic necrosis, pancreatitis, respiratory failure, or encephalopathy.

Laboratory.   Venous lactate >2 mmol/L is upper limit of normal, but symptoms are uncommon unless level is >5 mmol/ L. Other common laboratory findings are abnormal LFTs; increased anion gap; decreased chloride, albumin or bicarbonate; Computed tomography (CT) scan of abdomen may show steatosis.

Lactate measurement.   Patient should be hydrated and without vigorous exercise for 24 hr. Obtain venous blood without clenched fist using fluoride-oxalate (gray top) tube. Quality control is critical and erroneous results are common. Confirm results with second test.

Table 37. Treatment of Lactic Acidosis (IAS-USA; J AIDS 2002;31:257)

Lactate (mmol/L)	Symptoms	Intervention
<2	Yes or no	No interaction; other cause
2–5	Yes	Continue NRTIs, and follow lactate
5–10	Yes	D/C NRTIs: Use NNRTI/PI
>10	Yes	Medical emergency

Monitoring.   Not recommended in asymptomatic patients.

Frequency.   Estimated incidence is 0.08–0.8/100 pt-yr but much depends on the NRTI reviewed and the definition (AIDS 2000;14:F25; CID 2001;33:1931; AIDS 2000;14:2723; CID 2002;34:838; Expert Opin Pharmacother 2003;4:1321). Rank order of NRTIs: d4T/ddI > d4T > ddI > AZT > 3TC = ABC > TDF. Ribavirin is an added risk (Lancet 2001;357:280). Other risks are NRTI duration, female gender, obesity, and pregnancy.

Treatment.   D/C NRTI and give symptomatic care. Seriously ill patients may need IV bicarbonate, dialysis, hemofiltration and mechanical ventilation. Possibly effective agents include riboflavin (50 mg/day), antioxidants (vitamins C, E, and K), L-carnitine and thiamine (CID 2002;34:838) Resume with alternative NRTIs with low frequency of lactic acidosis (ABC, FTC, TDF) when lactate level is normal, and monitor levels. An alternative is an NRTI-sparing regimen.

Outcome.   Mortality correlates with lactate level: 5–10 mmol/L = 7%, 10–15 mmol/L = 30%, >15 mmol = 60–90% (CID 2002;34:838). The IAS-USA noted an overall mortality rate of 80% with lactate level >10 mmol/L and no mortality with <10 mmol/L. Response to treatment with NRTI withdrawal is slow owing to long half-life of mitochondrial DNA of 4–8 wk (NEJM 2002;346:811). Clinical recovery usually requires 4–28 wk and in one study required an average of 12 wk to return to normal (AIDS 2000;14:F25).

INSULIN RESISTANCE

Definition.   Impaired ability of insulin to increase muscle uptake of glucose and inhibit hepatic gluconeogenesis

Cause.   Associated with all PIs, but mechanism is unclear. IDV causes insulin resistance after single dose (AIDS 2002;16:F1); comparative data for other PIs is not available.

Monitoring.   Fasting blood glucose at baseline (pretreatment with PI) at 1–3 mo and at 3–6 mo intervals or more frequently if other risks or abnormal levels, and then annually. Diabetes is defined as FBS >126 mg/dL or >200 mg/dL 2 hr post 75 g glucose.

Treatment and Prevention.   In patients who are diabetic or diabetes prone (first-degree relatives) PI-sparing regimen may be preferred. With persistent increase in FBS, follow standard guidelines for management, usually starting with diet and exercise (Diabetes Care 2000;23[Suppl 1]:S32). If oral hypoglycemic agent necessary insulin-sensitizing agent (metformin or a thiazolidinedione) is often preferred. Monitor for hepatic dysfunction with LFTs q2 mo × 12 mo with thiazolidinediones and watch for lactic acidosis with metformin. ALT >2.5 × ULN at baseline contraindicates thiazolidinediones and elevated creatinine or lactate >2× ULN at baseline contraindicate metformin (Guidelines—IDSA and AACTG: CID 2003;37:613).

HYPERLIPIDEMIA

Definition.   PI-associated changes in lipid profile include increased total cholesterol, LDL cholesterol, and triglyceride resulting in a proatherogenic profile (JID 2004;189:1056; J AIDS 2000;23:35; Circulation 1999;100:700). Atazanavir is an exception. d4T is also implicated and EFV is implicated, but to a lesser extent. EFV and NVP are also associated with an increase in HDL. The effect appears greatest with RTV (AIDS 2000;14:51) and is nil with atazanavir. LPV/r results in a disproportionate increase in triglyceride levels that is largely due to the RTV component (AIDS; 2004;18:641). There is essentially no change in HDL cholesterol, and no PI has been shown to increase LDL cholesterol in persons without HIV infection (AIDS; 2004;18:641). Studies of NNRTIs show NVP and EFV are associated with increase in HDL cholesterol; results with EFV are contradictory. d_4T is associated with increased cholesterol and triglyceride.

Monitoring.   Fasting lipid profile at baseline, at 3–6 mo after starting or changing HAART and then ≥ annually or more frequently if risk factors and/or abnormal results. LDL = total cholesterol − HDL cholesterol − triglycerides/5; if triglyceride is >400 mg/dL, get direct LDL measurement.

Treatment.   National Cholesterol Education Program III guidelines are recommended (JAMA 2001;285:2486) with selec-

Table 38. National Cholesterol Education Program (NCEP) Recommendations—2002 (JAMA 2001;285:2486)

Risk	Lifestyle Changes LDL	Drug Therapy LDL	Goals of Therapy	
			LDL Cholesterol	Non-HDL Cholesterol
Coronary artery disease (CAD), other vascular disease (stroke, etc.) diabetes	>100**	>130	<70	<130
≥2 risk factors*	>130	>130–160	<100	<160
0 or 1 risk*	>160	>190	<160	<190

* Risk: smoking, hypertension (>140/90), HDL cholesterol <40 mg/dL, family hx early CAD in first-degree relative (male <55 or female <65).
** LDL cholesterol levels in mg/dL. Levels indicated are 2004 recommendations.

tive use of statins based on their interactions with protease inhibitors (Table 36 pg 98). For drug therapy, see Table 40.

Switch therapy— With high-risk profile, consider initiating or switching to PI-sparing regimen or ATV-based HAART

Life style changes— Reduced fat diet, weight loss, exercise, reduced ETOH. Note that smoking is a far greater risk for cardiovascular disease than protease inhibitors (NEJM 2003;349: 1993).

Table 39. Lipid-Lowering Drugs

Abnormality	Threshold	Intervention
Triglyceride	>500 mg/dL	Diet—low fat Gemfibrozil *or* fenofibrate
LDL cholesterol	Variable by risk: See Table 38	Pravastatin 20 mg* *or* Atorvastatin 10 mg* Fluvastatin, rasuvastatin, and cervistatin are other possible options (added by author)
High triglyceride *and* LDL cholesterol		Start with statin, Add fibrate after month 4**

* Doses are initial doses; escalate dose cautiously based on response.
** Both classes may cause rhabdomyolysis; use combination only when benefit exceeds risk.

FAT REDISTRIBUTION

Frequency.   40–50%

Cause.

PIs—evidence of causal role for visceral fat accumulation with increase in abdominal girth, lipomatosis, buffalo hump, and breasts.

d4T—Major agent implicated in peripheral fat loss with thinned extremities, buttocks, and buccal face fat.

NNRTIs—not implicated

Table 40. Methods to Assess Fat Redistribution: None Are Standard (JAIDS 2002;31:2570)

Method	Advantage	Disadvantage
CT scan	Gold standard	Expensive, radiation
MRI scan	Gold standard	Expensive
Anthropometric Waist: hip	Safe, portable inexpensive	Lacks specificity Requires training
Bioelectric impedance		Not validated (not recommended)
DEXA scan	Good for limbs, SAT	Not good for visceral fat
Ultrasound scan	Good for three-dimensional analysis	Limited published experience

DEXA, dual energy x-ray absorptiometry; MRI, magnetic resonance imaging.
* Conclusion is that none can currently be recommended.

Table 41. Treatment of Fat Redistribution

Treatment	Benefit	Other Benefit	Risk
Low-calorie diet	↓VAT	↓lipids	↓SAT
Exercise	↓VAT	↓TG ↑HDL	↓SAT
Metformin	↓VAT (?)	↓TG, ↓IR	↓SAT, LA
Thiazolidinediones	↓VAT ↑SAT	↓TR	Liver toxicity ↑TG
Growth hormone	↓VAT	↑HDL	↓SAT, ↑IR, diabetes
Testosterone physiologic	↓VAT	Improved	Men only
high dose	ND	—	↓HDL
Switch therapy	↓VAT (?)		Viral failure
Cosmetic surgery	—	—	Surgery risk

* VAT, visceral adipose tissue; SAT, superficial adipose tissue; TG, triglycerides; IR, insulin resistance; LA, lactic acidosis; ND, no data; HDL, high density lipoprotein cholesterol.

Lipoatrophy— D/C d4T; results with follow-up for 1–2 yr show no change or minimal change. For face thinning—injections of polylactic acid implants appear promising (AIDS 2003; 17:2471)

BONE DISEASE

Spectrum.   PI therapy is possibly associated with osteopenia in 22–50%, osteoporosis in 3–21%, and osteonecrosis in 0.1–1.3% but up to 4% with MRI screening; bone fractures are rare (Ann Intern Med 2002;137:17; AIDS 200;14:F63; AIDS 2001; 15:975). Risk of osteonecrosis is increased with increasing age, steroids, hyperlipidemia

Cause.   Unclear; role of antiretroviral therapy is unclear

Monitoring.   Not recommended

Diagnosis.   Usual presentation of osteonecrosis is joint pain especially of one or both femoral heads, which account for 85% of cases. Diagnosis is established by x-ray, MRI, or CT scan to detect osteonecrosis

Treatment.   If asymptomatic—follow with MRI q 3–6 mo for 1 yr, then q 6 mo to determine progression.

Osteonecrosis—surgical resection

Osteoporosis—evaluate for other risks including thyrotoxicosis, malabsorption, bed rest, severe weight loss, ETOH, medications (steroids, phenobarbital, pentamidine, ketoconazole. Rx— calcium, vitamin D, and weight bearing; if osteoporosis score is < -2.5 on DEXA scan: bisphosphonate

NUCLEOSIDE ANALOGS

AZT (Zidovudine)

Trade name: Retrovir (GlaxoSmithKline)

Forms.   100 mg caps and 300 mg tabs; IV vials with 10 mg/mL (20 mL); 300 mg in combination with lamivudine (3TC) as Combivir; 300 mg in combination with lamivudine (3TC) and abacavir (ABC) as Trizivir

Cost. $6.45/300 mg; $11.42/Combivir tab; $18.50/Trizivir tab

Financial assistance.   800-722-9294

Dose regimens

Standard— 200 mg PO tid or 300 mg bid or 1 Combivir bid or 1 Trizivir bid

Hepatic failure— standard dose

Renal failure—creatinine clearance ≤10 mL/min or dialysis 300 mg/day as single dose

Pregnancy— delivery—2 mg/kg/hr IV × 1 hr, then 1 mg/kg/hr IV until delivery; infant received 2 mg/kg PO q6h × 6 wk (MMWR 1994;43[RR-1]:1)

Advantages.   Extensive experience; established efficacy for preventing perinatal transmission (ACTG 076) and transmission following occupational exposure, for treatment of HIV-associated ITP and HIV-associated dementia; coformulated with 3TC ± ABC; no food effect

Disadvantages.   Need for bid dosing, toxicity (marrow suppression, asthenia, headaches, GI intolerance), TAMs with NRTI cross-resistance when continued in presence of virologic failure

Resistance— Thimadine analogue mutations (TAMs) include 41L, 67N, 70R, 210W, 215 Y/F, and 219 Q/E. The first to appear with dual nucleosides is usually 215 Y/F (J Infect Dis 2004;189: 862). The 184V mutation-associated with 3TC resistance delays resistance to AZT unless multiple TAMs are already present. Studies of acute HIV infection cases show the frequency of AZT resistance in newly infected persons in 1999–01 was 2–10% (NEJM 2002;347:385).

Pharmacology

Bioavailability— 60%; $T_{1/2}$serum: 1.4 hr; $T_{1/2}$ serum with renal failure: 1.4 hr; $T_{1/2}$ intracellular: 3 hr; CNS penetration: 60%

Elimination— metabolized to AZT glucuronide that is renally excreted as G-AZT

Note: AZT has superior CNS penetration compared with alternative nucleoside analogues; this may be an important factor in selection of drugs used in patients with dementia

Monitoring.   CBC q 3mo or more frequently with anemia or leukopenia

Note: nearly all patients develop clinically inconsequential macrocytosis within 4 wk of initiating AZT. The lack of macrocytosis should raise concern about compliance.

Side effects

Subjective complaints— headache, malaise, GI intolerance, insomnia, and/or asthenia—dose related and may resolve with continued treatment. GI intolerance is especially common and may improve with AZT administration with food and/or more frequent dosing.

Marrow suppression— with anemia and/or neutropenia. Frequency and severity related to dose, duration, and stage. Management: Discontinue with Hgb ≤7.5 g/dL or absolute neutrophil count (ANC) <750–1000/mm^3; alternative is coadministration of G-CSF or EPO, respectively.

Miscellaneous— *myopathy* with increased CPK; *hepatitis* with reversible increased transaminase levels; *cardiomyopathy* with reduced EF function by ECHO (association with AZT is unclear); *fingernail discoloration* (common and unimportant)

Lactic acidosis and hepatic steatotosis— class reaction; less common with AZT than with d4T (see pg 102)

Drug interactions

Marrow suppression— concurrent use with ganciclovir and other marrow-suppressing agents is usually contraindicated. Use with caution and monitor CBC carefully with dapsone, TMP-SMX, flucytosine, interferon, ribavirin, sulfadiazine, hydroxyurea, and amphotericin.

Miscellaneous— there is antagonism in vitro and in vivo when used in combination with d4T (stavudine). Concurrent use is contraindicated. Methadone increases AZT levels 30–40%; there is no effect on methadone levels (J AIDS 1998;18:435).

Pregnancy.   Category C

The National Cancer Institute reported in January 1997 that administration of AZT in doses 12–15 × those used in patients proved carcinogenic to the offspring of pregnant mice. A second study by GlaxoSmithKline using doses equivalent to those used in patients showed no carcinogenic potential in pregnant mice. NIH subsequently convened a panel to review these data. The unanimous conclusion was that the established benefits of AZT for preventing perinatal transmission outweigh the hypothetical risk. A subsequent report from France suggested mitochondrial toxicity with neurologic sequelae in children exposed to AZT in utero (Lancet 1999;354:1084) This prompted a large-scale evaluation of 20,000 infants exposed to AZT in utero that showed no evidence of immunologic, oncogenic, cardiac, or neurologic consequences (NEJM 2000;343:805).

ddl (Didanosine)

Trade name: Videx and Videx EC (Bristol-Myers-Squibb)

Forms.   *Buffered tabs:* 25, 50, 100, 150, and 200 mg. The 200 mg tabs are formulated for once daily dosing (400 mg qd).

Videx EC is an enteric-coated capsule without buffer for once daily administration: 125, 200, 250, and 400 mg. Advantages of Videx EC: 1) once daily administration, 2) possibly improved GI tolerance (less diarrhea), and 3) avoidance of buffer-related drug interactions.

Cost.   Buffered tabs: 200 mg—$5.63; Videx EC 400 mg cap—$11.20

Financial assistance.   800-272-4878

Dose regimens

Standard—administration on an empty stomach

	Buffered Tabs[a]	Videx EC Caps
Food	>1 hr before or >2 hr after meal	>1/2 hr before or 2 hr after meal
>60 kg dose	200 mg bid or 400 mg qd	400 mg qd
<60 kg dose	125 mg bid or 250 mg qd	250 mg qd
with TDF	250 mg qd	250 mg qd

[a] Tabs must be chewed thoroughly or crushed and dissolved in water.

Renal failure

Renal failure	>60 kg	<60 kg
CrCl 30–59	200 mg/d	125 mg/d
CrCl 10–29	125 mg/d	100 mg/d
CrCl <10	125 mg/d	75 mg/d

A concern with renal failure is Na^+ (11.5 mEq/tab) and Mg^{++} (15.7 mEq/tab). With hemodialysis or peritoneal dialysis: 25% standard dose

Hepatic failure—standard dose

Advantages.   Extensive experience; once daily dosing; avoid TAMs

Disadvantages.   Need for dosing on empty stomach; restricted use of co-administered ribivarin; need for dose adjustment when given with TDF; toxicity profile—peripheral neuropathy, pancreatitis, lactic acidosis, GI intolerance

Resistance.   Most important is 65R, which causes cross-resistance to ABC and TDF

Pharmacology

Bioavailability—30–40%. Food decreases bioavailability by 55%. Should take all formulations on empty stomach

$T_{1/2}$ serum—1.6 hr; $T_{1/2}$ renal failure—3.1 hr; $T_{1/2}$ intracellular—25–40 hr; CNS penetration—20%

Elimination—renal: 50%

Monitoring.   Amylase q 1–2 mo was at one time advocated, but utility of this practice for preventing severe pancreatitis is unclear; and the frequency of this complication with ddI appears to have significantly and inexplicably decreased during the HAART era. Most important is to warn patient of symptoms of pancreatitis and peripheral neuropathy.

Side effects

Peripheral neuropathy—in 5–12% related to dose and duration. Management: discontinue ddI or reduce dose.

Pancreatitis—in 1–9%; frequency appears to be less in HAART era for unexplained reasons. Risk increases with history of pancreatitis, advanced HIV, alcoholism, and concurrent medications that cause pancreatitis and with concurrent d4T and/or hydroxyurea. Management of pancreatitis—discontinue ddI.

Gastrointestinal intolerance—Videx EC is better tolerated; methods to improve tolerance of buffered tabs are to dissolve tabs in ice water or apple juice or try powder form.

Miscellaneous—marrow suppression, hyperuricemia, hepatitis, and rash

Lactic acidosis and hepatic steatosis—class adverse effect (see pg 102)

Drug interactions

Interactions from buffer in ddI formulations—drugs requiring gastric acidity should be given 2 hr before or 2 hr after ddI—indinavir, ritonavir, atazanavir, delavirdine, fluoroquinolones, dapsone, ketoconazole, itraconazole, and tetracyclines. (These interactions are not seen with Videx EC.)

Atazanavir—buffered ddI reduces ATV AUC 87%—use Videx EC but must separate dosing because ATV requires food and ddI requires empty stomach

Pancreatitis and neuropathy—drugs that cause pancreatitis should be used with caution: pentamidine, ethambutol, and alcohol. Drugs that cause peripheral neuropathy should be used with caution or avoided: cisplatin, ddC, d4T, disulfiram, ethionamide, INH, phenytoin, vincristine, hydralazine, metronidazole (long-term use only), and glutethimide.

Tenofovir—results in 40–60% increase in ddI AUC and may increase risk of peripheral neuropathy or pancreatitis. Recommendation is to use dose of 250 mg/day, but no recommendation for dose adjustment for those <60 kg has been made.

Methadone—methadone reduces AUC of ddI by 60%; ddI has no effect on methadone. (J AIDS 2000;24:241)

Ribavirin—increases intracellular ddI levels and may cause toxicity—avoid (Antivir Ther 2004;9:133)

Pregnancy.   Category B; ddI combined with d4T should be avoided in pregnancy because of three deaths ascribed to lactic acidosis.

ddC (Dideoxycytidine, Zalcitabine)

Trade name: Hivid (Hoffman-LaRoche)
   Forms.   0.375 and 0.75 mg tabs
   Cost. $2.84/0.75 mg tab

Financial assistance.   800-282-7780

Dose regimen

Standard—0.75 mg tid

Renal failure—creatinine clearance >50 mL/min—0.75 mg tid; 10–40 mL/min—0.75 mg bid; <10 mL/min—0.75 mg q 24 h; dialysis—no data

Hepatic failure—standard dose

Advantages.   None

Disadvantages.   Minimal evidence of antiviral effect; requirement for tid dosing; high rate of peripheral neuropathy

Pharmacology

Bioavailability—85%

$T_{1/2}$ serum—1.2–2 hr; $T_{1/2}$ intracellular—3 hr; CNS penetration—20%

Elimination—renal excretion 70%

Monitoring.   Warn patient of symptoms of peripheral neuropathy

Side effects

Peripheral neuropathy—17–31%, related to dose and duration. Management: Discontinue; patients with mild symptoms or symptoms that have resolved may be treated with half dose.

Miscellaneous—stomatitis, aphthous ulcers, pancreatitis, hepatitis

Drug interactions

Peripheral neuropathy—drugs that cause peripheral neuropathy should be avoided or used with caution—ddI, d4T, cisplatin, disulfiram, ethionamide, INH, phenytoin, vincristine, glutethimide, gold, hydralazine, and metronidazole

d4T (Stavudine)

Trade name: Zerit (Bristol-Myers-Squibb)

Forms.   15, 20, 30, and 40 mg caps; oral solution 1 mg/mL (200 mL); Zerit XR 100, 75 mg caps

Cost. $5.55/15 mg cap; $5.77/20 mg cap; $6.13/30 mg cap; $6.25/40 mg cap

Financial assistance.   800-272-4878

Dose regimen

Renal failure

Wt.	Creatinine clearance		
	>50 mL/min	26–50 mL/min	<10 mL/min and dialysis
>60 kg	40 mg bid	20 mg q bid	20 mg qd
<60 kg	30 mg bid	15 mg q bid	15 mg qd

Hepatic failure—standard

Advantages.   Well-tolerated; once daily dosing, no food effect

Disadvantages.   Long-term toxicity (lipoatrophy, peripheral neuropathy, lactic acidosis, risk of TAMs)

Pharmacology
Bioavailability—86% (not influenced by food)

$T_{1/2}$ serum—1 hr; $T_{1/2}$ renal failure—8 hr; $T_{1/2}$ intracellular—3.5 hr; CNS penetration—30–40%

Elimination—renal 50%

Monitoring.   Warn patient of symptoms of peripheral neuropathy; warn of symptoms of pancreatitis if given concurrently with ddI

Side effects   d4T is well tolerated early in course of treatment, but long-term consequences may be severe, especially when combined with ddI

Peripheral neuropathy—15–21%, related to dose and duration

Miscellaneous—pancreatitis, hepatitis, neutropenia

Class adverse effects—mitochondrial toxicity with lactic acidosis ± hepatic steatosis; major cause of lipoatrophy (see pg 102)

Drug interactions
d4T-AZT interaction—stavudine shows pharmacologic antagonism with AZT, presumably because of competition for intracellular phosphorylation. Concurrent use is contraindicated

Peripheral neuropathy—drugs that cause peripheral neuropathy should be avoided or used with caution: Ethionamide, ethambutol, INH, phenytoin, vincristine, glutethimide, gold, hydralazine, long-term metronidazole. Concurrent use with ddI should be done with caution because of increased risk of lactic acidosis, pancreatitis and peripheral neuropathy; this combination is contraindicated in pregnancy because of three deaths attributed to lactic acidosis in pregnant women.

Methadone—concurrent use with methadone shows little effect on d4T levels and no effect on methadone levels

Monitoring.   Warn patient about pancreatitis and peripheral neuropathy, especially with ddI

Pregnancy.   Category C; combination of ddI + d4T should be avoided in pregnancy because of three deaths ascribed to lactic acidosis

3TC (Lamivudine)

Trade name: Epivir (GlaxoSmithKline)

Forms.   Oral solution with 10 mg/mL; 150 mg and 300 mg tabs lamivudine (3TC); 150 mg + AZT 300 mg as Combivir; 150 mg + AZT 300 mg and ABC 300 mg as Trizivir; 300 mg + ABC 600 mg as Epzicom; 100 mg tabs for treatment of hepatitis B

Cost. $5.52/150 mg tab; $11.04/300 mg tab; $11.42/Combivir tab and $18.50/Trizivir tab

Financial assistance.   800-722-9294

Dose regimen

Standard for HIV—150 mg po bid or 300 mg qd; Epzicom — 1 tab qd

Standard for hepatitis B—100 mg/day × 52 wk

Renal Failure, CrCl Levels	HBV (mg/day)*	50 qd or 150 mg qod
>50 mL/min	100	150 bid
10–50 mL/min	100	150 qd
<10 mL/min	10–15	50 qd or 150 mg qod
Dialysis	10	25–50 qd

* Loading dose of 100 mg with CrCl >15 mL/min; <15 mL/min use 35 mg loading dose.
** Loading dose of 150 mg.

Hepatic failure—HIV: Standard dose

Hepatitis B virus is inhibited by lamivudine (NEJM 2004;350: 118); treatment of patients who were co-infected with HIV and HBV show significant reduction in HBV DNA concentrations (Ann Intern Med 1996;125:705). A 1-yr trial with 100 mg/day vs placebo showed that patients with chronic HBV infection had reduced rates of progression to fibrosis, enhanced elimination of HBV DNA, and clearance of HBVe Ag (NEJM 1998;339:61). Resistance by HBV is predicted owing to mutations on the YMDD gene (J Clin Virol 2000;24:173; CID 1999;28:11032; Lancet 1997;349:20). Alternatives are to add tenofovir or adofovir, which are effective vs. lamivudine-resistant strains.

Resistance. High-level resistance with 184V evolves within 3–4 wk with 3TC treatment in non-suppressive regimens. This mutation increases susceptibility to AZT, d4T, and TDF, and decreases susceptibility of ABC (when combined with TAMs) and ddI

Advantages. Well-tolerated; no food effect, potential for once daily therapy, co-formulated with AZT (Combivir) and AZT/ABC (Trizivir) and ABC; 184V mutation slows AZT resistance; active vs 11BV

Disadvantages. Rapid evolution of high-level resistance when given in presence of virologic failure; relatively rapid evolution of resistance by HBV; may cause HBV flare if discontinued

Pharmacology. Oral bioavailability—86%; $T_{1/2}$ serum— 3–6 hr; $T_{1/2}$ intracellular—12 hr; CNS penetration—10%; elimination—renal 71%.

Side effects. Generally well tolerated. Minor: Headache, nausea, diarrhea, abdominal pain, and insomnia

Drug interactions. None

Pregnancy. Category C

FTC (Emtricitabine)

Trade name: Emtriva (Gilead)

Forms. 200 mg cap; 200 mg + tenofovir 300 mg as Truvada

Cost. $10.10/200 mg cap (FTC) $26/Truvada tab

Financial assistance. 800-272-4878

Dose regimen

200 mg qd; Truvada − 1 tab qd

Renal failure—CrCl 30–49 mL/min—200 mg q 48 h; 15–29 mg/min—200 mg q 72 h; < 15 mL/min—200 mg q 96 h

Renal failure Truvada—CrCl 30–49 mL/min—1 tab q 48 h; < 30 mL/min: Not recommended

Hepatic failure—No dose change

Resistance.   M184 mutation evolves rapidly with nonsuppressive regimen and confers high level resistance

Advantages.   Potent, well tolerated, no food effect, once daily coformulated with tenofovir

Disadvantages.   Rapid evolution of 184 V mutation with resistance; may cause HBV flare if discontinued

Pharmacology.
Bioavailability—93% absorbed; no food effect; Half life—10 hrs; 39 hr intracellular; Elimination—Primarily renal

Monitoring.   None

Side effects.   Occasional GI intolerance, headache, asthenia rash or hyperpigmentation

Class adverse reactions—Lactic acidosis has not been reported

HBV—May cause resistance to FTC and 3TC; monitor for hepatitis B flare with HBV chronic hepatitis if discontinued

Drug interactions.   None

Pregnancy.   Category B

ABC (Abacavir)

Trade name: Ziagen (GlaxoSmithKline)

Form.   300 mg tabs; oral suspension with 20 mg/mL; 300 mg + 3TC 150 mg + AZT 300 mg as Trizivir; 600 mg + 3TC as Epzicom

Cost. $7.41/300 mg tab; $18.50/Trizivir tab; $27/Epzicom

Financial assistance.   800-722-9294

Dose regimens.
Standard—300 mg PO bid; Epzicom − 1 tab qd
Renal failure—standard dose
Liver failure—no data

Resistance.   ABC selects for 74V and to a lesser extent 65R; these each reduce ABC activity 2–4-fold and cause cross-resistance with ddI. ABC resistance usually requires multiple mutations; 3 TAMs plus 184 predict ABC resistance (Antivir Ther 2004;9:37)

Advantages.   No food effect; once daily dosing; low potential for mitochondrial toxicity; co-formulated with AZT/3TC (Trizavir) and 3-TC; avoids TAMs; no dose adjustment for renal or hepatic failure; potential for once daily therapy

Disadvantages.   Hypersensitivity reactions

Resistance.   Selects primarily for 74V and to a lesser extent for 65R. Significant resistance requires multiple mutations (Antiviral Ther 2004;9:37)

Pharmacology

Bioavailability—83%, food—no effect, $T_{1/2}$—1.5 hr; intracellular $T_{1/2}$—3.3 hr; CNS levels are 27–33% of serum levels

Elimination—81% metabolized by alcohol dehydrogenase and glucuronyl transferase; metabolites are excreted in urine; 16% is recovered in stool, and 1% is unchanged in urine (metabolism does not involve cytochrome P-450 enzymes)

Side effects

Hypersensitivity reaction—a serious side effect reported in 5% of ABC recipients with fatalities in 0.03% (3/10,000) (Clin Ther 2001;23:1603). Clinical features are fever (usually >39°C), fatigue, malaise, GI symptoms (nausea, vomiting, diarrhea, abdominal pain), cough, and skin rash (maculopopular or urticarial) and may be difficult to distinguish from flu (Clin Infect Dis 2002;34:1137). The rash is noted in about 70% and nearly all patients have fever. Lab tests may show elevated liver function tests and CPK and lymphopenia. Rechallenge may be lethal. About 90–95% of these reactions occur within 6 wk of initiating treatment; median time of onset in one series was 9 days (Lancet 2002;356:1423). Susceptibility to this reaction has been associated with HLA-DR7 and HLA-DO3 halotypes (Lancet 2002;359: 727; PNAS 2004;101:4180), but screening for this genetic pattern is not yet practical. These reactions should be reported to the Abacavir Hypersensitivity Registry at 800-270-0425. Patients taking ABC should be warned of this reaction and should stop taking ABC or report to their provider if they develop suggestive symptoms. A concern is unnecessary discontinuation because of common intercurrent illnesses. For this reason, we generally ask the patient to contact the provider to review symptoms before discontinuation; in some cases, the patient reports to clinic for administration under observation—this will predictably lead to a reaction if caused by ABC hypersensitivity. Caution is needed because after discontinuation, rechallenge may cause an anaphylactic-like reaction with hypotension, bronchospasm, and/or renal failure, sometimes resulting in death (AIDS 1999;13:999). Treatment is supportive; steroids and antihistamines are not helpful.

Miscellaneous—nausea, vomiting, malaise, headache, diarrhea, or anorexia

Lactic acidosis and steatosis—class reaction, but this is unusual with ABC

Monitoring. Warn patient regarding hypersensitivity reaction as a systemic reaction with fever, GI symptoms, and rash seen primarily in the first 6 wk of treatment. Warn not to rechallenge.

Drug interactions. Alcohol increases ABC AUC 41% (AAC 2000;283:1811). Significance is unclear.

Pregnancy. Category C

TDF (Tenofovir)

Trade name: Viread (Gilead)

Form. 300 mg tab; 300 mg + emtricitabine 200 mg as Truvada

Cost. $13.60/300 mg tab; $27/Truvada

Financial assistance. 800-272-4878

Dose regimens. 300 mg qd; Truvada 1 tab qd

Renal failure—Cr Cl 30–50 mL/min—300 mg qod; 10–30 mL/min—300 mg q 4 day, <10 mL/min—300 mg q 7 day; hemodialysis—300 mg q 7 day,

Hepatic failure—No change

Resistance. Susceptibility is decreased in the presence ≥3 TAMs that include 41L and 210W and with the T69 insertion (Antimicrob Ag Chemother 2004;48:992). The 65R mutation also causes resistance unless 184V is also present.

Advantages. Well-tolerated, once daily, low pill burden, does not reduce TAMs, low potential for mitochondrial toxicity, active vs HBV including 3TC-resistant strains (JID 2004;189: 1185); co-formulated with FTC

Disadvantages.   Difficulty in using with reduced renal function (see below); may cause acute HBV flare if discontinued

Pharmacology.

Bioavailability—25% fasting and 40% with food; take with meal, especially a high-fat meal

$T^{1/2}$—12–18 hr; intracellular: 10–50 hr

Elimination—Renal

Monitoring.   Creatinine, urinanalysis, serum K, and serum phosphorus in patients with pre-existing renal disease or concurrent nephrotoxic drugs

Side effects.   Main concern is nephrotoxicity with Fanconi syndrome primarily in patients who are predisposed by concurrent nephrotoxic drugs or pre-existing renal disease, which may be subtle with normal serum creatinine. (Note recommendation to use half dose with a creatinine clearance of 30–49 cc/mL)

Miscellaneous GI intolerance, hepatitis, neutropenia, and elevated amylase

Class ADR—Lactic acidosis is rare (not reported)

Drug interactions.

ddI: TDF increases ddI levels 40–60% with potential to increase rates of ddI-associated peripheral neuropathy, pancreatitis, and lactic acidosis. Recommendation for this combination is to reduce the standard ddI dose to 250 mg/day

Pregnancy.   Category C

PROTEASE INHIBITORS

Atazanavir (ATV) Trade name: Reyataz (Bristol)

Form.   150 and 200 mg caps

Cost. $14.49/200 mg cap

Dose.   400 mg (2 caps) qd or ATV 300 mg qd (2 150-mg caps) + RTV 100 mg qd; take with food

Renal failure—Standard

Hepatic failure—Child Pugh score 7–9—use 300 mg qd; Child Pugh score >9—avoid ATV

Tenofovir or efavirnz co-administration—Use ATV 300 mg qd + RTV 100 mg qd

Resistance.   Signature resistance mutation is 50L, which is often accompanied by 71V; these mutations increase in vitro activity of ADV, IDV, LPV, NFV, RTV, and SQV, but clinical significance is unknown (JID 2004;189:1802). ATV activity is reduced by >3 PI class mutations: 46IL, 32AFTS, 84VAC, 90M (Antimicrob Ag Chemother 2003;47:1324).

Advantages.   Potency comparable to EFV (BMS 034) and LPV/r (with boosting) (AI 424-043); once daily dosing; boosts well with RTV; minimal lipid effect even with RTV boosting; low pill burden; unique resistance mutation (50L)

Disadvantages.   Increased indirect bilirubin which is medically inconsequential but may cause jaundice; multiple drug interactions including drugs that reduce gastric acidity; food requirement

Pharmacology.   Requires gastric acid for absorption. Food increases AUC 70%

Serum half life—7 hr

Metabolism—Inhibits and is substrate for P 450 3 A4. Metabolized and metabolites are excreted by liver

Side effects.

Increased indirect bilirubin due to UGT 1A1—no medical consequences but jaundice in about 7%

Cardiac—Prolonged QTc and PR interval—use with caution with other drugs that prolong QTc

GI/Liver—Occasional GI intolerance and increased transaminases

Class adverse reactions—Does not cause lipid changes but implicated in fat redistribution and diabetes (see pg 103–107)

Monitoring.   FBS at baseline and at 1–3 mo; then annually or more frequently if clinically indicated.

Drug interactions.

Drugs contraindicated for concurrent use—Astemizole, bipridil, cisapride, ergotamine, indinavir, irinotecan, levostatin, and mi-

dazolam, pimozide, *protein pump inhibitors,* rifampin, simvastatin, St John's wort, terfenadine

Drugs that required dose adjustment:
- Rifabutin RBT 150 mg qod or $3 \times$/wk
- Clarithromycin: Clari—half dose
- Oral contraceptives: Estradiol AUC increased 48% and
  norethindrone AUC increased 110%—use lower dose or
  alternative
- Statins—pravastatin preferred; atorvastatin—use lowest
  dose
- Anticonvulsants—ATV decreased by carbamapezine, phe-
  nobarbitol, and phenytoin; use with caution
- Sildenafil—maximum dose is ≤25 mg/24 hr, vardenafil
  ≤2.5 mg/24 hr, and <2.5 mg/72 hr when ATV is boosted
  with RTV
- Diltiazem: Use half-dose diltiazem and monitor EKG
- H_2 receptor antagonists: Separate dosing by 12 hr
- Antacids and buffered meds—Give 2 hr before or 1 hr after
  ATC;
- Buffered ddI—use ddI EC (Videx EC) but separate dosing
  by ≥ 2 hr
- Tenofovir—Use standard dose TDF and boosted ATV

PI-NNRTI combinations—See Table 36

Pregnancy   Category B. It is not known if the increased
indirect bilirubin will increase risk of neonatal hyperbilirubi-
nemia.

Fosamprenavir Trade name: Lexiva (Glaxo SmithKline)

Forms.   700 mg tab

Cost. $10.48/700 mg tab

Financial assistance.   800-722-9294

Dose regimen

1400 mg bid; 700 mg + RTV 100 mg bid or 1400 mg + RTV
200 mg qd

Renal failure—No dose adjustment

Hepatic failure—Child Pugh score 5–8: 700 mg bid; score >
9; not recommended. (Note: RTV boosting should not be used
with hepatic impairment)

Advantages. Should replace APV except when used in combination with LPV/r, no food effect, boosts well with RTV, relatively few drug interactions, favorable resistance profile to preserve PI options, once daily, less effect on lipids compared to other PIs

Disadvantages. Once daily regimen, but this is not recommended for PI experienced patients

Resistance. Primary mutation is I 50 V, which confers LPV/r resistance and I 84 V—a multi-PI resistant mutation

Pharmacology
Absorption—Not effected by food
T1/2: 7.7 hrs.
Elimination—APV is inhibitor and inducer of P450 3A4

Adverse reactions
Skin rash—12–33% of patients; discontinuation required in <1%. Use with caution in patients with sulfonamide sensitivity.

GI intolerance—Reported in up to 40%, but severe in only 5–10%. Rate of GI intolerance was similar to that of NFV in NEAT except for more diarrhea with NFV

Hepatitis—ALT levels >5x ULN in 6–8%

Lipids—Minimal impact of FPV alone unless boosted with RTV (see pg 103–107)

Drug interactions. Identical to those described with APV except for some PI/NNRTI combinations (see Table 36)

Pregnancy Category C. Data on safety and pharmacokinetics are inadequate to recommend in pregnancy not advocated for treatment experienced patients; ATV is preferred for use in combination with LPV/r; high rate of skin rash.

Saquinavir. Trade name: Fortovase and Invirase (Hoffman-LaRoche)
Forms. 200 mg caps (soft gel capsules as Fortovase and hard gel capsules as saquinavir mesglate or Invirase); 500 mg Invirase tab expected January 2005
Cost. 200 mg caps at $2.50 (Invirase); 200 mg caps at $1.33 (Fortovase)

Financial assistance.   800-282-7780

Dose regimen

Standard—SQV is nearly always used in combination with RTV. Initially, it was thought that Fortovase would entirely supplant the use of Invirase owing to better bioavailability. However, subsequent work has shown that the pharmacokinetic profile of Invirase is comparable to that of Fortovase when each is given with ritonavir, and Invirase is better tolerated. Invirase has consequently become the favored formulation and the major issue is the dose:

1) SQV/r* 1000 mg/100 mg bid
2) SQV/r* 1600 mg/100 mg qd or 12000/100 qd
3) SQV/r* 2000 mg/100 mg qd (with Invirase 500 mg caps)
4) SQV/r 400 mg/400 mg bid

*SQV may be Fortovase or Invirase, but most prefer Invirase.

 Renal failure—standard

 Hepatic failure—standard; use with caution

Resistance.   Most common is 90M, which reduces phenotype sensitivity 3-fold, and the most important is 48V, which reduces sensitivity 30-fold. Like most other PIs, ≥2 mutations or protease gene at codons 10, 46, 82, 84, and 90 confer resistance

Advantages when combined with RTV.   Extensive experience; extensive experience with good pharmacokinetics and tolerance in pregnancy; potency comparable to EFV in Focus trial (but inferior to LPV/r in MaxCMin2)

Disadvantages.   GI intolerance (less with Invirase); high pill burden

Pharmacology

Bioavailability—4% for Invirase when taken with high-fat meal to promote absorption; Fortovase is better absorbed with three-fold increase in AUC; food increases bioavailability. When taken with RTV, the dual PI regimens eliminate need for food and difference in absorption. $T_{1/2}$ serum—1–2 hr without RTV boosting; CNS penetration—poor

Elimination—96% biliary excretion via cytochrome P-450, 1% in urine

Side effects.   Dose-related GI intolerance with nausea, abdominal pain, and diarrhea in 20–30% (Fortovase) or 5–10% (Invirase); headache; hepatitis; hypolgycemia with type 2 diabetes (Ann Intern Med 1999;181:980)

Class adverse effects—hyperlipidemia, fat accumulation, and insulin resistant hyperglycemia (see p 103–107)

Monitoring—fasting lipid profile (cholesterol, LDH, HDL, triglycerides) and fasting blood glucose at baseline and at 3–6 mo; frequency of subsequent measurements depends on test results and other risk factors

Drug interactions

Drugs that are contraindicated for concurrent use—astemizole, cisapride, simvastatin, lovastatin, pimozide, rifampin, ergot alkaloids, midazolam, St. John's wort, simvastatin terfenadine, and triazolam

Drugs affected by saquinavir—Atorvastatin levels ↑ 450%—start with 10 mg/d; sildenafil—≤25 mg/48 hr; tadalafil—≤10 mg/72 hr; Vardenafil—≤2.5 mg/72 hr

Drugs that reduce saquinavir levels—nevirapine, phenobarbital, phenytoin, dexamethasone, carbamazepine, and garlic; rifampin and rifabutin (see below)

Drugs that increase levels of saquinavir—drugs that inhibit cytochrome P450 increase levels of saquinavir, including ketoconazole, itraconazole, fluconazole, ritonavir, indinavir, nelfinavir, delavirdine and grapefruit juice

Rifampin/rifabutin—rifampin reduces SQV levels by 80%, and rifabutin reduces SQV levels by 40%; these drugs should not be used concurrently unless SQV is combined with RTV, a rifampin-containing regimen (MMWR 2000;49:185).

Combination with PI or NNRTIs   (See Table 36)

Indinavir Trade name: Crixivan (Merck)

Forms.   200, 333 and 400 mg capsules
Cost. $6.21/400 mg cap
Financial assistance.   800-850-3430
Dose regimen
Standard—800 mg q8h in fasting state or with a light, non-fat meal. Patient should take >48 oz fluid/day to reduce fre-

quency of nephrolithiasis. Store in original container with desiccant. Regimens commonly used to increase IDV levels and to avoid the inconvenience of q8h dosing is 1) IDV 400 mg bid + RTV 400 mg bid or 2) IDV 800 mg bid + RTV 100–200 mg bid. The 400/400 mg regimen may be difficult for patients to tolerate due to the RTV dose; the 800/100–200 mg regimen may cause a higher rate of nephrolithiasis.

Renal failure—standard

Hepatic failure—600 mg q8h

Resistance.   Major protease resistance mutations are 46I/L, 82 A/F/T, and 84V; minor mutations are at codons 10, 20, 24, 32, 36, 54, 71, 73, 77, and 90 (Topics in HIV Med 2003;11:94). Resistance usually requires ≥ 3 mutations. These multiple mutations are usually associated with class resistance

Advantages.   Extensive experience including long-term follow-up (≥ 6 yr for Merck 035)

Disadvantages.   Need for q8 hr dosing (unless boosted) risk of nephrolithiasis and need for large fluid intake; GI intolerance; sicasydrome and alopecia; PI cross-resistance

Pharmacology

Bioavailability—absorption is best with fasting state or with a light meal that does not contain fat; food is not an issue when taken with RTV

$T_{1/2}$ serum—1.5–2 hr

Excretion—metabolized, especially hepatic glucuronidation and P-450-dependent pathways. Urine shows 5–12% unchanged drug and metabolites.

Levels—Peak levels correlate with risk of nephrolithiasis and trough levels correlate with antiviral efficacy; great individual variation in pharmacokinetics (JAIDS 2002;29:374), suggesting possible role for therapeutic drug monitoring (Antimicrob Ag Chemother 2001;45:236).

Side effects

Renal stones & nephritis—IDV may cause nephrolithiasis or interstitial nephritis. Most common side effect is renal stones composed of indinavir precipitates with crystals that may be seen on urinalysis in up to 60% of IDV recipients. Nephroliasis with renal colic, flank pain, and hematuria ± renal insufficiency is reported at 8/100 pt-yr (Arch Intern Med 2000;162:1493). Incidence correlates with peak serum levels of indinavir; hydration and urinary pH are other factors. Should take 48 oz fluid daily, preferably at time of IDV administration. Management options are to reduce IDV dose (efficacy not established), increase hydration, therapeutic drug monitoring, or switch to alternative therapy. Most do the latter. Indinavir may also cause interstitial nephropathy with proteinuria and renal failure (CID 2000;34: 1033).

Elevated indirect bilirubin—inconsequential increase in indirect bilirubin to >2.5 mg/dL without other changes in liver function tests in 10–15%

Skin, hair, & nails—IDV is associated with alopecia involving all body hair (NEJM 1999;341:618); paronychia and ingrown toenails; and the sicca syndrome with dryness of eyes, skin, and mucous membranes.

Miscellaneous—hepatitis with increased transaminase levels, headache, nausea, vomiting, diarrhea, metallic taste, fatigue, insomnia, blurred vision, dizziness, rash, thrombocytopenia

Class adverse effect—lipodystrophy, insulin resistant hyperglycemia and hyperlipidemia. Insulin resistance was shown in healthy volunteers with IDV given 4 wk (AIDS 2001;15:F11). This effect is greater than with other PIs (AIDS 2004;18:641) (see p 103–107).

Monitoring—serum creatinine and urinanalysis at 3- to 6-mo intervals. Fasting lipid profile (cholesterol, HDL, LDL, triglyceride) and blood glucose at baseline and at 3–6 mo; frequency of subsequent tests depends on initial results and concurrent risks

Drug interactions

Combinations with PIs and NNRTIs: See Table 36

rifampin and rifabutin decrease levels of indinavir, and indinavir increases levels of rifabutin. Concurrent use with rifampin is contraindicated; rifabutin should be reduced to half dose (150 mg/day or 300 mg 2–3×/wk), and IDV is increased to 1000 mg tid.

Drugs that are contraindicated for co-administration—astemizole, cisapride, rifampin, simvastatin, lovastatin, St John's wort, midazolam, terfenadine, ergotamines, triazolam

ddI—buffered ddI given concurrently decreases indinavir

absorption; these drugs should be given ≥2 hr apart or use Videx EC

Miscellaneous—ketoconazole and itraconazole increase IDV levels 70%; decrease IDV dose to 600 mg q8h. Concurrent use with voriconazole has no significant effect on either IDV or voriconazole. Clarithromycin levels increase 53%—no dose change. Ethinyl estradiol levels increase—no dose change. Anticonvulsants (phenobarbital, phenytoin, carbamazepine) may decrease IDV levels. Sildenafil (Viagra) levels increase 4 ×; maximum sildenafil dose is 25 mg/48 hr; maximum tadalafil dose is 10 mg/72 hr; maximum vardenafil dose is 2.5 mg/72 hr. Grapefruit juice decreases IDV 26%. Methadone levels are unchanged.

Pregnancy.   Category C

Ritonavir Trade name: Norvir (Abbott)

Form.   100 mg caps; 600 mg/7.5 mL PO

Cost.   New AWP price is $10.71/100 mg; price to Medicaid, ADAP, and other federal or state payors is $2.14/100 mg cap

Patient assistance program.   800-659-9050

Dose regimen

Standard—600 mg bid PO; dose-escalation regimen days 1–2: 300 mg bid; days 3–5: 400 mg bid; days 6–13: 500 mg bid; day ≥14: 600 mg bid. Virtually no one uses RTV as a sole PI, but it is used to boost other PIs (daily dose usually 100–200 mg/day) or to boost companion PI and achieve antiviral activity of RTV (≥400 mg bid). See Table 36 for combination.

Renal failure—standard

Hepatic failure—standard dose; use with caution

Resistance.   (Relevant only when used in doses likely to achieve antiviral effect). Major mutations are 82 A/F/T/S and 84V; minor mutations are at codons 10, 20, 32, 33, 36, 46, 54, 71, 77, and 90. Cross-resistance with IDV is nearly complete

Advantages of RTV boosting.   Boosts all PIs except NFV; pharmacologic benefit of boosting is established and now considered standard of care for most PI-based HAART

Disadvantages.   GI intolerance of RTV which is dose-related; hepatotoxicity

Pharmacology

Bioavailability—not been determined

$T_{1/2}$ serum—3–5 hr

Excretion—hepatic metabolism by cytochrome P450 mechanism. Ritonavir induces its own excretion so that therapeutic levels are achieved with the graduated-dose regimen.

Side effects

GI intolerance—the major limiting side effect and sufficiently severe to require discontinuation of full-dose RTV in 30% (J AIDS 2000;23:236); intolerance is dose-related and often improves with treatment over 1 mo

Hepatotoxicity—RTV appears to cause drug-induced hepatitis more frequently than other PIs (JAMA 2000;238:74). The lower doses used with PI combinations appear to cause less hepatotoxicity.

Miscellaneous—Circumoral and peripheral paresthesias.

Class ADRs—fat redistribution, insulin resistant hyperglycemia, and hyperlipidemia. RTV appears to cause more elevation of LDL cholesterol and triglyceride than other PIs (J AIDS 2002; 31:257; J AIDS 2000;23:261; JAMA 2000;23:236; NEJM 2003;349: 199) (See pages 103–107).

Monitoring.   Fasting lipid profile (cholesterol, LDL, HDL, triglycerides) and fasting blood glucose at baseline and 3–6 mo; frequency of subsequent tests depends on initial test results and concurrent risks.

Drug interactions

Drugs that are contraindicated for current use—astemizole, amiodarone, bepridil, cisapride, encainide, ergot alkaloids, flecainide, lovastatin, midazolam, pimozide, propafenone, quinidine, simvastatin, terfenadine, St John's wort, triazolam, and voriconazole

Voriconazole—AUC of voriconazole is decreased 82% with RTV 400 mg bid. Avoid combination with full-dose RTV, but implication for low doses used for boosting is unclear

Atorvastatin—RTV/SQV increase AUC of atorvastatin 450%—use atorvastatin in low dose (10 mg/d) or use pravastatin or fluvastatin

Miscellaneous—Other interactions include increase in levels of clarithromycin (CID 1996;23:6) (no dose change); induction of hepatic glucuronyl transferase and CYP1A2 activity results in reduced levels of ethinyl estradiol—alternative methods of birth control should be used. Methadone levels are decreased 36% but decrease in R isomer is slight; no dose adjustment for methadone is likely. Desipramine levels are increased 145%; decrease desipramine dose. Buffered ddI reduces absorption of RTV, and the two drugs should be taken ≥2 hr apart or use Videx EC. Rifabutin levels are increased 4×, and the rifabutin dose should be reduced to 150 mg qod and RTV is standard dose.

Concurrent use with other PIs—See Table 36.

Pregnancy.   Category B

Nelfinavir Trade name: Viracept (Agouron Pharmaceuticals)

Form.   250 mg and 625 mg tabs; 50 mg/g oral powder

Cost. $2.52/250 mg tab

Dose.   750 mg PO tid or 1250 mg bid with meal

Renal failure.   Standard

Hepatic failure.   Standard dose

Resistance.   The signature resistance mutation is 30N, which does not cause cross-resistance with other PIs. Another resistance mutation is 90M, which does cause cross-resistance

Advantages.   Extensive experience; one of best-tolerated PIs, extensive experience, and well-tolerated in pregnancy; protease resistance mutation at 30N does not cause cross-resistance with other PIs; new 625 mg tab reduces pill burden from 10/d to 4/d

Disadvantages.   Less potent versus HIV in several comparative trials (EFV superior in ACTG 384, LPV/r superior in M98-863 and FPV superior in NEAT); food requirement; diarrhea; lack of significant boosting with RTV.

Pharmacology

Bioavailability—20–80%; food, especially fatty food, increases absorption 2–3× $T_{1/2}$ serum: 3.5–5 hr

Excretion—hepatic cytochrome P-450, only 1–2% found in urine and up to 90% is found in stool primarily as oxidative metabolites

Side effects

In therapeutic trials, only 28 of 696 (4%) discontinued nelfinavir owing to side effects, usually because of diarrhea; 10–30% experience loose stools, and most respond to imodium.

Class adverse reaction—lipodystrophy; insulin resistant hyperglycemia; hyperlipidemia. The severity and frequency of hyperlipidemia appears to be less that that with ritonavir or lopinavir (J AIDS 2002;31:257) (see p 103–107).

Monitoring. Fasting lipid profile (cholesterol, LDL, HDL, triglycerides) and fasting blood glucose at baseline and at 3–6 mo; frequency of subsequent tests depends on results of baseline tests and associated risk factors.

Drug interactions

Drugs that must be avoided for concurrent use—cisapride, astemizole, midazolam, terfenadine, rifampin, St John's wort, ergot alkaloids, and triazolam

Rifampin/rifabutin—rifampin reduces nelfinavir levels substantially and should not be given concurrently; rifabutin is not problematic for nelfinavir, but rifabutin levels increase 3-fold so that the rifabutin dose should be reduced to half (150 mg/d or 300 mg 2–3×/wk).

Interactions with other PIs—interactions are less pronounced compared with other agents in this class (see Table 36):

Indinavir—IDV 1200 mg bid + NFV 1250 mg bid

Ritonavir—RTV 400 mg bid + NFV 500–750 mg bid

Saquinavir—SQV (Fortovase) 800 mg tid or 1200 mg bid + NFV 1250 mg bid or 750 mg tid

Amprenavir—APV 800 mg tid + NFV 750 mg tid (limited data)

Nevirapine—standard doses both drugs

Efavirenz—standard doses both drugs

Lopinavir/ritonavir—no data

Delavirdine—DLV 600 mg bid + NFV 750 mg tid

Pregnancy. Class B

Amprenavir (APV). Trade name: Agenerase (GlaxoSmith-Kline)

Note: This drug is largely antiquated by the availability of Fosamprenavir, which is the APV prodrug that permits a substantial reduction in pill burden. A possible exception is APV + LPV/r, which permits these drugs together

Form. 50 mg caps; 150 mg soft gel caps; 15 mg/mL oral solution

Cost. $1.60/150 mg cap

Financial assistance. 800-722-9294

Dose standard. 1200 mg bid (eight 150 mg caps) given with or without food, but avoid high-fat meal; oral solution 1400 mg bid

Renal failure—standard dose

Hepatic failure—moderate disease 450 mg bid; severe cirrhosis 300 mg bid

Pharmacology

Bioavailability—89%, AUC decreased 21% by concurrent high fat meal

$T_{1/2}$—7–9.5 hr

Elimination—hepatic metabolism CYP 3A inhibition is <RTV and comparable with IDV and NFV

Side effects Major reasons to discontinue APV are GI intolerance and rash

GI intolerance—nausea (15%), diarrhea (14%), vomiting (5%)

Rash—6–11%; this drug is a sulfonamide, but prior reactions attributed to sulfonamides do not appear to be a contraindication

Oral solution—contains 55% propylene glycol and is contraindicated in pregnancy, renal failure, hepatic failure and in patients receiving atabuse. Patients receiving this formulation should not consume ETOH

Miscellaneous—headache 6%, oral paresthesias 28%. APV contains large amounts of vitamin E (1744 units/day with 2400 mg daily dose); this with vitamin E supplement could produce bleeding diathesis.

Class adverse reactions—lipodystrophy, insulin resistant diabetes, and hyperlipidemia (see pg 103–107)

Monitoring. Fasting blood lipids (cholesterol, LDL, HDL, triglycerides) and blood glucose at baseline, at 3–6 mo and then annually or more frequently if clinically indicated.

Drug interactions

Drugs contraindicated for concurrent use—astemazole, bepridil, cisapride, ergotamines, lovastatin, midazolam, rifampin, terfenadine, St John's wort, simvastatin, triazolam

Drugs that must be given with caution—amiodarone, carbamazepine, clozapine, lidocaine, phenobarbital, phenytoin, quinidine, tricyclics, warfarin, oral contraceptives (use alternative methods)

Combination with other PIs and NNRTIs—See Table 36

Rifampin/rifabutin—rifampin reduces APV AUC 82% and should not be used concurrently. Rifabutin decreases APV AUC 15%, and APV increases RFB AUC 20%; use RFB 150 mg/day or 300 mg 2–3×/wk + APV standard dose.

Miscellaneous—clarithromycin increases APV AUC 32%; use standard dose of both drugs. Ketoconazole increases APV AUC 44%; dose implications are unclear.

Pregnancy.   Category C

Lopinavir/ritonavir (LPV/r). Trade name: Kaletra (Abbott)

Form.   Capsules with 133 mg lopinavir + 33 mg ritonavir; oral solution with 80 mg LPV + 20 mg RTV/mL

Cost. $3.90 per 133/33 mg cap

Financial assistance.   800-659-9050

Product information.   800-633-9110

Dose

Standard—400/100 mg bid (3 caps bid) or 800/200 mg qd (ARV-naive patients only) with food

Renal failure—standard dose

Hepatic failure—standard dose

Resistance.   Major mutations have not been identified and patients who fail LPV/r initial therapy usually have no resistance mutations. Resistance in vitro correlates with multiple mutation that confer PI class resistance LPV/r

Advantages.   Antiretroviral potency with comparable or superior antiviral activity compared to alternative agents in all clinical trials; durability with 5-year follow-up (AIDS 2004;18:775); co-formulated with RTV; generally well-tolerated

Disadvantages.   Food requirement; probable need for bid dosing for optimal activity; diarrhea as a common side effect; lipid effect; limited experience in pregnant women

Pharmacology

Bioavailability: 80% with food; 48% with fasting. The RTV "boost" increases the mean steady-state concentration of LPV by 15–20-fold

$T_{1/2}$ 5–6 hr

Elimination—metabolized by P450 CYP 3A4 isoenzymes. Less than 3% excreted in urine

Side effects

Gastrointestinal—most common, especially diarrhea that can usually be managed with loperamide (Imodium). For nausea, the oral solution may be better tolerated

Miscellaneous—hepatotoxicity in 10–12%; asthenia; oral solution has 42% ETOH, giving possible disulfiram reaction

Class adverse reactions—lipodystrophy, insulin-resistant hyperglycemia, and hyperlipidemia. The greatest lipid effect is increased triglycerides, which is largely attributed to the ritonavir component (AIDS 2004;18:641) (see pg 103–107)

Monitoring.   Fasting blood lipids (cholesterol, LDL, HDL, triglycerides) and blood glucose at baseline and at 3–6 mo and annually; more frequently if clinically indicated

Drug interactions

Drugs contraindicated for concurrent use—astemizole, cisapride, ergot derivatives, midazolam, lovastatin, pimozide, simvastatin, St. John's wort, terfenadine, flecainide propafenone, rifampin and triazolam. Phenytoin; phenobarbital, and carbamazepine.

Drugs that require dose change—rifabutin 150 mg qod + LPV/r standard dose

Clarithromycin—AUC clarithromycin increased 77%; reduce clarithromycin dose in renal failure

Oral contraceptives—Ethinyl estradiol AUC decreased 42%—use alternative birth control

Erectile dysfunction—Sildenafil—limit to 2.5 mg/72 hr; tadalafil—limit to 2.5 mg/72 hr; vardenafil—limit to 2.5 mg/72 hr

Atorvastatin—AUC atorvastatin increased 450%; use lowest possible dose (10 mg/d) or use alternative, such as fluvastatin or pravastatin

Drugs to use with caution—ketoconazole levels increased 3×—limit ketoconazole dose to ≤200 mg/d; anticonvulsants may decrease LPV levels—monitor anticonvulsant level. Do not give with qd dose.

Dose adjustments with PIs and NNRTIs   (See Table 36)

Pregnancy.   Category C

NON-NUCLEOSIDE REVERSE TRANSCRIPTASE INHIBITORS

Nevirapine Trade name: Viramune (Roxane Labs)

Form. 200 mg tabs; 50 mg/5mL oral solution

Cost. $6.01/200 mg tab

Dose

Standard—200 mg qd ("lead in" ×2 wk), then 200 mg po bid unless rash precludes standard dose. If therapy is interrupted >7 days, then 200 mg dose should be restarted. May be given with or without food. Monitor liver function tests, especially during first 8 wk.

Renal failure—standard

Hepatic failure—consider empiric dose reduction

Resistance. Virologic failure associated with rapid and high-level resistance with mutations 100I, 103N, and/or 188 C/I. There is cross-resistance with DLV; cross-resistance with EFV is variable, but complete and high-level with 103N

Advantages. Extensive experience; 2NN study showed antiviral activity similar to EFV (Lancet 2004;363:1253); few drug interactions; extensive experience in pregnancy (but most of it is with a single dose at delivery); no food effect

Disadvantages. High rates of potentially fatal hepatotoxicity primarily with initial therapy in women with CD4 counts > 250/mm^3; high rates of rashes including Stevens—Johnson and TEN; single mutation may eliminate use of the entire class

Pharmacology

Bioavailability—average is 93%; food has no effect, CSF penetration—45% of serum levels.

$T_{1/2}$—25 hr

Excretion—biotransformed by hepatic cytochrome P-450 enzymes. Nevirapine induces P-450, reducing its own half-life so that the half-life of 45 hr with early therapy is reduced to 25 hr.

Side effects

Hepatotoxicity—There are two forms—the most important is a serious hepatitis associated with fever, rash and/or eosinophilia. This usually occurs in the first 18 wk of therapy, primarily the first 6 wk, the rate is especially high at 11% in women who receive NVP as initial therapy with a baseline CD4 count > 250/mm^3. This reaction may be fatal even with prompt discontinuation of NVP. The second form of hepatitis is an elevation of the ALT that is usually asymptomatic and usually reversible, even with continuation of NVP. (Lancet 2001;357:687).

Rash—seen in about 17%; usual rash is maculopapular and erythematous with or without pruritus located on the trunk, face, and extremities. Most rashes are seen during the first month; 7% of all patients require discontinuation of the drug. Indications to discontinue therapy are severe rash or rash accompanied by fever, blisters, mucous membrane involvement, conjunctivitis, edema, arthralgias, or malaise. (Lancet 1998;351:567).

Miscellaneous side effects include fever, nausea, and headache.

Monitoring.   Monitor ATL and AST every 2 wk × 1 mo, then monthly × 3, and then every 3 mo. Patients who develop a rash or fever which receiving NVP should have LFTs. There is no assurance that this monitoring will be effective in preventing severe NVP hepatotoxicity.

Drug interactions.   NVP, like rifampin, induces P450 CYP3A4 isoenzymes resulting in enhanced metabolism of drugs metabolized by this mechanism. Clinically significant drug interactions are less frequent with NVP than with PIs and other NNRTIs. For example, few drugs are considered contraindicated for concurrent use, and most known drug interactions require only modest changes.

Not recommended for concurrent use—rifampin, voriconazole and ketoconazole

Drugs that show interactions—*rifabutin* decreases NVP levels 16%: no dose change; *clarithromycin* levels decrease 30% and NVP levels increase 26%: no dose change; *ethinyl estradiol* levels decrease 20%: use alternative method. *Methadone* levels decrease 60%, making dose elevations necessary for methadone (Clin Infect Dis 2001;33:1595): titrate methadone dose by symptoms or avoid the combinations anti-seizure agents (phenobarbital, phenytoin, carbamazepine) have not been studied.

PI combinations   See Table 36

Pregnancy.   Class C

Single-dose regimen at delivery is highly effective in preventing perinatal transmission, especially when combined with AZT given in the last trimester (NEJM 2004;351:217). However, the single NVP dose has been associated with NVP resistance mutations in 19% (NEJM 2004;351:229)

Delavirdine (DLV). Trade name: Rescriptor (Agouron)

Form.   100 and 200 mg tabs

Cost. $1.62/200 mg tab

Dose standard.   400 mg po tid. Food—minimal effect; ddI and antacids—take 1 hr apart

Renal failure—standard dose

Hepatic failure—consider dose reduction with severe liver disease

Pharmacology

Bioavailability—85%; CSF penetration poor (CSF; plasma = 0.02)

$T_{1/2}$—5.8 hr

Elimination—metabolized by cytochrome P-450 CYP 3A enzymes; delavirdine inhibits CYP 3A to increase its own levels and levels of IDV, NFV, SQV; 51% excreted in urine and 44% in feces

Side effects

Rash—18%; 4% require discontinuation; rash is diffuse, maculopapular, and red and on upper body. Stevens-Johnson syndrome reported and usually lasts 2 wk and resolves despite continuation of DLV. Discontinue if rash and fever, mucous membrane involvement, accompanying symptoms of swelling or arthralgias

Miscellaneous—headache

Monitoring.   Warn regarding rash reaction

Drug interactions

Drugs contraindicated for concurrent use—terfenadine, rifampin, rifabutin, ergot derivatives, astemizole, cisapride, midazolam, triazolam, H_2 blockers, proton pump inhibitors, simvastatin, lovastatin

Drugs with interactions requiring dose changes—clarithromycin levels increased 100%, and DLV levels increased 44%; adjust dose with renal failure; DLV may increase levels of dapsone, wafarin, and quinidine; for sildenafil, do not exceed 25 mg/48 hr; take antacids and buffered ddI >1 hr apart or use Videx EC

Drugs that decrease levels of delavirdine—carbamazepine, phenobarbital, phenytoin, rifabutin, and rifampin

PI combinations See Table 36

Pregnancy.   Category C

Efavirenz (EFV). Trade name: Sustiva (DuPont)

Form.   50, 100, 200 mg caps; 600 mg tab

Cost. $16.17/600 mg tab

Patient assistance program.   800-272-4878

Dose standard.   600 mg PO hs

Renal failure—standard dose

Hepatic failure—consider empiric dose reduction

Resistance.   The 103N mutation is selected and confers high-level class resistance. Other RT mutations associated with resistance are 100I, 106M, 108I, 181C/I, 188L, 190S/A, and 225H.

Advantages.   EFV is superior or comparable to all comparitors in clinical trials for initial therapy; durable antiviral activity with 5-yr follow-up data; once-daily therapy; low pill burden; no food effect; may be used with rifampin

Disadvantages.   Single mutation confers high-level class resistance; high rate of CNS toxicity that is usually self-limited; teratogenic risk in first trimester

Pharmacology

Bioavailability—40–45% with or without food; high-fat meals increase absorption 50% and should be avoided. Serum levels are highly variable (AIDS 2001;15:71; Antimicrob Ag Chemother 2004;48:979)

$T_{1/2}$—40–55 hr; CSF 0.25–1.2% of serum levels

Elimination—metabolized by P-450 CY 3A4 isoenzymes; 14–34% excreted in urine as glucuronide metabolites and 16–61% excreted in stool

Side effects

CNS—noted in 52%, usually resolve in 2–3 wk and require discontinuation in 2–5%. Symptoms include confusion, abnormal dreams, dizziness, impaired concentration, and "depersonalization." Less common are hallucinations, somnolence, insomnia, amnesia, and euphoria. Patients should be warned, EFV is given at bedtime to reduce symptoms that are noted with the first dose and may be confounded with alcohol or other psychoactive drugs. Cause is unknown.

Rash—about 15–27% develop rash that is usually morbilliform and usually does not require discontinuation. Rashes that are blistering or show desquamation are noted in 1–2%; Stevens-Johnson syndrome is reported in 1 of 2200 treated patients. Rash sufficiently severe to require discontinuation occurs in about 2% compared with NVP at 7%.

Hepatotoxicity—transaminase levels increase to $>5 \times$ ULN in 2–8% (Hepatology 2002;35:182).

Lipid abnormalities—Lipid changes show increases in cholesterol, but there are conflicting data about the critical issue of whether it is HDL or LDL cholesterol; most studies show increases in HDL and LDL cholesterol with variable effects on triglycerides (J AIDS 2002;31:257; CID 2000;31:1266; J AIDS 2000;24:310).

Teratogenicity—teratogenic in primates, so pregnant women should strictly avoid EFV, and women of childbearing potential should be warned. There is a single case report of a myelomingocele in a child born to a mother who was taking EFV during the first trimester (Arch Intern Med 2002;162:355).

Monitoring

CNS—patients must be warned of CNS effects that are anticipated with most patients, are usually apparent after the first dose, and usually resolve after 3 wk. Dose administration at bedtime is only partially effective in restricting symptoms to sleep time owing to long half-life of the drug. Particular caution is advised in patients with a history of mental illness, drug addiction, or alcoholism and those receiving psychoactive drugs

Women of childbearing potential—warn of teratogenic effect of EFV and the need for adequate contraception, preferably with two forms. EFV should be avoided by women who are contemplating pregnancy, and during the first trimester.

Lipodystrophy—EFV is commonly associated with an increase in cholesterol, including an increase in HDL. Effects on triglyceride levels, glucose levels, and fat redistribution are unknown; some authorities recommend monitoring analogous to that for PI recipients, i.e., fasting blood lipids and blood glucose at baseline and at 3–6 mo; subsequent tests depend on results of initial tests, risk factors, and results of ongoing trials.

Drug interactions

Drugs contraindicated for concurrent use—astemizole, midazolam, triazolam, cisapride, and ergot alkaloids

Drugs that decrease EFV levels—phenobarbital, phenytoin, and carbamazepine

Rifampin/rifabutin—EFV reduces rifabutin levels 35%; no effect of RFB on EFV levels. Use EFV 600 mg/day + RFB 450 mg qd or 600 mg 2–3×/wk, EFV standard dose. Rifampin decreases EFV levels 25%—use EFV 800 mg qd

Other interactions—when clarithromycin levels decrease 39% and the rate of rash reaction is increased; use alternative. When levels of ethinyl estradiol are increased 37%, use alternative. When methadone levels decrease, monitor for withdrawal; interaction with coumadin suspected; monitor anticoagulation

PI combinations(See Table 36)

Pregnancy. Category C

Efavirenz should be avoided during pregnancy and should be given only with due caution to women with child-bearing potential, remembering that its interaction with birth control pills may render them ineffective. The basis for the concern in the first trimester is: 1) Neural defects in 3 of 20 gravid cytomolgus monkeys; 2) a report of a myelomeningocele in a child born to a woman taking EFV at the time of conception (Arch Intern

Med 2002;162:355); 3) The Antiretroviral Pregnancy Registry shows 4 of 142 live births with EFV exposure had birth defects; and 4) the 2003 package insert includes 3 cases of neural tube defects. Note that exposure in the second and third trimester should be safe.

FUSION INHIBITORS

Enfuvirtude (T20) Trade name: Fuscon

Form.   Packaged as 30-day supply kit with 60–90 mg single-use vials of enfuvirtude and 60 vials sterile water for injection and 60–3 mL reconstitution syringes and 60–1 mL syringes for SC injection. The kit can be stored at room temperature, but once the drug is reconstituted it should be refrigerated and used within 24 hr

Cost.   60–90 mg vials @ $2,082

Regimen.   1 mL (90 mg) SC bid, rotating injection sites
Renal failure—Standard dose
Hepatic failure—Standard dose

Resistance.   Mutations at the gp41 receptor site confer resistance including gp 41 codons 36, 38, 40, 42, 43, and 45

Advantages.   Potent antiviral activity; resistance in untreated patients is nil; well-studied in Toro 1 and 2 (NEJM 2003; 348:2175; NEJM 2003;348:2168)

Disadvantages.   Requirement for bid SC injections; local hypersensitivity reactions at infection sites; need for a concurrent active drug for sustained activity

Pharmacokinetics
Bioavailability—84% from injection sites
Metabolism—Unknown
Elimination—Metabolic pathway is unknown.

Side effects.
Local—Injection site reactions are very common with erythema in 30%, pruritis in 60%, and induration in 90%; nodules and cysts are noted in 26%. These reactions appear to be local hypersensitivity reactions and are sufficiently severe to require discontinuation in only about 3%.

Other ADR's—The rate of bacterial pneumonia is increased 5-fold for reasons that are unclear. Rare ADRs include generalized rash, nausea, vomiting, chills, fever, hypotension, increased transaminase neutropenia, eosinophilia, Guillaun Barre syndrome, and elevated amylase. A causal relationship with many of these reactions is unclear.

Drug interactions.   None

Pregnancy.   Category B

8—Management of Complications

Table 42. Management of HIV-Associated Complications

Opportunistic Infections (from Bartlett JG and Gallant J. 2004 Medical Management of HIV Infection. Baltimore: Johns Hopkins University, Division of Infectious Diseases, 2001) (see www.hopkins-aids.edu)

	Preferred Regimen(s)	Alternative Regimen(s)	Comments
		FUNGAL INFECTION	
PNEUMOCYSTIS CARINII **Acute infection**	Trimethoprim 15–20 mg/kg/d + sulfamethoxazole 75–100 mg/kg/day PO or IV × 21 days in 3–4 divided doses (typical oral dosage is 2 DS tid)	Trimethoprim 15 mg/kg/day PO + dapsone* 100 mg/d PO × 21 days Pentamidine 4 mg/kg/day IV × 21 days (usually reserved for severe cases) Clindamycin 600 mg IV q8h or 300–450 mg po q6h + primaquine* 30 mg base/d PO × 21 days Atovaquone 750 mg suspension PO with meal bid × 21 days Trimetrexate 45 mg/m² IV day plus folinic acid 20 mg/m² PO or IV q6h	*Options:* In a comparative trial (ACTG 108) TMP-SMX, trimethoprim-dapsone, and clindamycin-primaquine were equally effective in patients with mild-to-moderate PCP (Ann Intern Med 1996;124:792) *ADRs to TMP-SMX:* Intolerance to TMP-SMX is noted in 25–50%, primarily skin rash ± fever (Lancet 1991;338:431)

143

Table 42. (continued)

	Preferred Regimen(s)	Alternative Regimen(s)	Comments
		FUNGAL INFECTION	
PCP (prophylaxis): See p. 50			*Steroids:* Patients with moderately severe or severe disease (PO$_2$ <70 mmHg or A- a gradient >35 mmHg) should receive corticosteroids (prednisone 40 mg po bid × 5 days, then 40 mg qd × 5 days, then 20 mg/day to completion of treatment). Side effects include CNS toxicity, thrush, H. simplex infection, tuberculosis, and other OIs (J AIDS 1995;8:345)
ASPERGILLOSIS Invasive pulmonary infection (NEJM 2002:355;423)	Voriconazole 6 mg/kg IV q 12hr ≥1 wk, then 200 mg bid. Note interactions between PIs and voriconazole	Amphotericin B 1.0-1.4 mg/kg/day Itraconazole 200 mg PO bid with food (capsules) or 100-200 mg bid with empty stomach (liquid) Itraconazole 200 mg IV bid × 4, then 200 mg IV qd Amphotec 5 mg/kg/day IV Abelcet 5 mg/kg/day IV AmBisome 5 mg/kg/day IV Caspofungin 70 mg IV × 1, then 50 mg IV/day	*Predisposing factors:* Corticosteroids: decrease or stop if possible; neutropenia: G-CSF and avoid 5-FC *Recommendations* based on IDSA guidelines (MMWR 2002:51; RR-6) and updated by comparative trial that favored voriconazole for invasive aspergillosis based on cure rates and survival (NEJM 2002:355;423) *Lipid Ampho B:* preparations include Abelcet, Amphotec, and AmBisome. Advantage is reduced nephrotoxicity and less infusion related reactions. Best studied is AmBisome, but high dose often required and AWP cost is >$1000/d *Trials:* Best results with voriconazole (NEJM 2002:356;423). Response rate to voriconazole (200-400 mg/day) was

			Comments
CANDIDA Oropharyngeal (thrush) initial infection (see HIV Clin Trials 2000;1: 47; CID 2000:32: 662)	Clotrimazole oral troches 10 mg 5×/day or Nystatin susp 4-6 ml qid or pastilles 4-5×/d or Fluconazole 100 mg po	*Fluconazole refractory:* Amphotericin B 0.3-0.5 mg/kg/day IV Itraconazole‡ 200 mg/day oral suspension *Relapsing disease:* Chronic fluconazole if recurrences are frequent or disabling	*Duration:* Treat until symptoms resolve (usually 10-14 days) *Azoles:* Fluconazole is superior to ketoconazole with better efficacy, fewer drug interactions, more predictable absorption, but higher price. Itraconazole—efficacy comparable with fluconazole but more drug interactions (Am J Med 1998;104:33) *Resistance:* In vitro resistance is most common with prior azole exposure, late stage HIV infection, and non-albicans species Some report high rates of response (48/50) to fluconazole despite in vitro resistance (JID 1996;174:821). Doses up to 800 mg/day may be tried
Maintenance (optional or as needed: see "Comments")	Clotrimazole (previously stated dose) Fluconazole 100 mg/day PO or 200 mg 3×/wk	Itraconazole‡ 200 mg (tabs)/day or 100 mg PO suspension qd Ketoconazole‡ 200 mg/day PO Nystatin (previously stated dose)	*Indications for chronic Rx:* Recurrent debilitating thrush *Non-response:* Endoscopy to confirm if not done previously. Options: 1) Increase fluconazole dose; 2) Use alternative azole (vori or itra) or alternative class—IV caspofungin, IV ampho B *Resistance:* Concerns with continuous treatment with fluconazole are azole resistance by Candida species, drug interactions, and cost. Risks for azole resistant Candida infections are prolonged azole exposure and low CD4 count (JID 1996;173:219)

Table 42. (continued)

	Preferred Regimen(s)	Alternative Regimen(s)	Comments
		FUNGAL INFECTION	
Candida prophylaxis	Not recommended		
Candida vaginitis (MMWR 2002:51 (RR-6)	Intravaginal miconazole suppository 200 mg × 3 days or cream (2%) × 7 days Clotrimazole cream (1%) × 7–14 days or tabs: 100 mg qd × 7 days or 100 mg 2/day × 3 days or 500 mg × 1 Fluconazole 150 mg po × 1	Itraconazole 200 mg po bid × 1 day or 3 days	*Fluconazole:* Fluconazole is superior to clotrimazole in preventing relapses of thrush but risks azole resistance *Relapse:* Most patients will relapse within 3 mo after therapy if treatment is discontinued in absence of immune reconstitution. Options are treatment of each episode or maintenance *Duration:* May require continuous treatment to prevent relapse: fluconazole 50–100 mg/day PO, or fluconazole 200 mg/wk PO *OTC:* Clotrimazole and miconazole (both cream and 100 mg tabs) are available over-the-counter *Prophylaxis:* Weekly fluconazole (200 mg) appears to be effective without risk of azole resistance in women with CD4 count >300/mm³ (Ann Intern Med 1997;126:689) *Overview:* Treatment is identical with and without HIV infection (MMWR 47(RR-1):78, 1998)
Candida esophagitis Initial infection	Fluconazole 100–200 mg/ day po; up to 400 mg/ day × 2–3 wk Itraconazole‡ 200 mg oral suspension/day	*Fluconazole-refractory:* • Caspofungin 70 mg IV × 1, then 50 mg IV/d • Ampho B 0.3–0.7 mg/kg/day	*Azoles:* Fluconazole is clinically superior to ketoconazole as initial treatment *Relapse rate* is 84% within 1 yr in absence of immune reconstitution and prophylaxis after therapy *Azole resistance:* Candida causing esophagitis are infrequently azole-resistant (CID2002:30:749)

			appears superior to Amphotericin B (CID 2001;33:1529; AAC 2002;46:451) Voriconazole is equivalent to fluconazole, and may be superior with fluconazole-resistant strains (CID 2001;33:447; AAC 2002;46:451) *Chronic Rx:* Consider maintenance therapy in patients with recurrent esophagitis, although probability of resistance is increased (JID 1996;173: 219)
Candida Maintenance if recurrent or disabling	Fluconazole 100–200 mg/day po	Ketoconazole 200 mg/day PO Itraconazole 200 mg/day PO (tabs) or 100 mg/day oral solution	
CRYPTOCOCCAL MENINGITIS Initial treatment (CID 2000: 30:710)	Amphotericin B 0.7 mg/kg/day IV + flucytosine 100 mg/kg/day po × 14 days. Consolidation: fluconazole 400 mg/d × 8–10 wk or until CSF culture is sterile. *Management of intracraneal pressure:* 1. Focal CNS signs or obtunded—MRI or CT scan before LP, which may show contraindication to LP 2. Normal OP—medical management and LP at 2 wk for culture, etc. 3. OP >250 mmH₂O—CSF drainage until pressure <200 or 50% initial value; repeat LP daily until nil 4. Elevated pressure persists—lumbar drain or VP shunt	Fluconazole 400 mg/day PO × 6–10 wk. Itraconazole‡ 200 mg PO tid × 3 days, then 200 mg PO bid (see "Comments") Fluconazole 400 mg/day PO plus flucytosine 100 mg/kg/day PO Amphotericin B 0.7 mg/kg/day IV × 14 days (without flucytosine) *Consolidation alternative:* Itraconazole 200 mg po bid *Renal failure or Ampho B intolerance:* Lipid formulation at 4 mg/kg/d IV and Flucytosine 25 mg/kg qid po × 2 wk	*Initial regimen:* Amphotericin B is preferred for initial treatment, but total dose before fluconazole maintenance is arbitrary *Consolidation:* Usual tactic is to change to oral fluconazole at 14 days or to make this decision based on CSF cultures at 10–14 days *Initial Rx with fluconazole:* Fluconazole is acceptable as initial treatment only for patients with normal mental status. Other favorable prognostic findings are cryptococcal antigen <1:32 and CSF WBC >20/mm³ *Dx:* Cryptococcal antigen is nearly always detected in CSF but less useful in monitoring response; sensitivity of serum antigen is 95%, usually at titer >1:2048, but it is useless in monitoring response *Azoles:* Itraconazole: ACTG 159 showed itraconazole (400 mg/day) was as effective as fluconazole (400 mg/day) with 8 wk treatment after initial treatment with amphotericin B 0.7 mg/kg/day ± flucytosine × 14 days (NEJM 1997;337:15)

Table 42. (continued)

	Preferred Regimen(s)	Alternative Regimen(s)	Comments
		FUNGAL INFECTION	
			Fluconazole may be used in doses up to 800 mg/day for salvage therapy
			5-FC: Flucytosine + amphotericin B are superior to amphotericin B alone (NEJM 337:15, 1997); flucytosine + fluconazole are also superior to fluconazole alone but show high rates of reactions (CID 1998;26:1362; CID 1994;19:74)
Maintenance	Fluconazole 200 mg/day PO	Amphotericin B 1 mg/kg 1 ×/wk Fluconazole: May increase maintenance dose to 400 mg/day, or Itraconazole‡ 200 mg bid	*Rules:* Life-long maintenance treatment unless there is immune reconstitution with CD4 > 100–200 /mm³ > 6 mo. initial therapy completed and pt is asymptomatic (CID 2003;36:1329) *Itraconazole:* Disadvantage is poor CNS penetration *Fluconazole* maintenance at 200 mg/d is superior to amphotericin B (NEJM 326:793, 1992) and superior to itraconazole at 200 mg PO/day (CID 1999;28:291)
Prophylaxis (see "Comments")	Not generally recommended	Fluconazole 200 mg PO/day Itraconazole 200 mg/PO/day or 100 mg oral suspension/day	*Efficacy:* Efficacy has been shown for all patients with CD4 counts <50/mm³, but concerns are that *Cryptococcus* is infrequent (8–10%), possible azole-resistant *Candida,* possible drug interactions, and cost

			Comments
CRYPTOCOCCOSIS WITHOUT MENINGITIS (pulmonary, disseminated, or antigenemia)	Fluconazole 200 mg PO bid Indefinitely unless immune reconstitution	Itraconazole‡ 200 mg PO bid	*LP:* All patients with positive cultures or stain evidence of cryptococcosis should have lumbar puncture to exclude meningitis *Antigenemia:* Chest x-ray, LP, urine and blood culture. If no focus identified and antigenemia persists treat with fluconazole (CID1996;23:827)
Maintenance (see "Comments")	Fluconazole 200 mg/day PO	Itraconazole‡ 200 mg/day or 100 mg oral suspension/day Amphotericin B 0.6–1 mg/kg IV weekly or 2 ×/wk	Need for maintenance treatment is not established
HISTOPLASMOSIS Disseminated, initial treatment	Amphotericin B 0.5–1.0 mg/kg/day IV × ≥ 7–14 days Itraconazole‡ 300 mg PO bid × 3 days, then 200 mg PO bid or 100–200 mg oral suspension bid (mild-moderately severe disease) AmBisome IV 3–5 mg/kg/day × 3–10 days	Fluconazole 1600 mg po × 1, then 800 mg/day × 12 wk, then 400 mg/day (Am J Med 1997;103:223)	*Initial Rx:* Itraconazole may be used for initial treatment of mild to moderate histoplasmosis without CNS involvement or it may be used for maintenance after induction with amphotericin B (Am J Med 1995;98:336) *Itraconazole levels:* Should verify itraconazole levels (San Antonio Lab 210-567-4131) *Other azoles:* Fluconazole is less active than itraconazole and may require doses of 600–800 mg/day for primary or maintenance therapy; ketoconazole is not recommended
Maintenance	Itraconazole‡ 200 mg PO bid	Amphotericin B 1.0 mg/kg 1 ×/wk Fluconazole 400 mg PO/day	*Azoles:* Efficacy of itraconazole is established (Ann Intern Med 1993;118:610) and is superior to fluconazole (Am J Med 1997;103:223) *Immune reconstitution:* Data are inadequate to provide guidelines for discontinuation of maintenance therapy owing to immune reconstitution

Table 42. (continued)

	Preferred Regimen(s)	Alternative Regimen(s)	Comments
		FUNGAL INFECTION	
Prophylaxis	Itraconazole‡ 200 mg PO/day	Fluconazole 200 mg po/day	*Indication:* Consider in endemic area with CD4 <100/mm³, especially if at high risk owing to occupation (work with soil) or hyperendemic rate (>10 cases/100 pt-yr) (MMWR 199;948(RR-10):24)
COCCIDIOIDOMYCOSIS Initial treatment	Amphotericin B 0.5 mg/kg/day IV × ≥ 8 wk: total dose 2–2.5 g Fluconazole 400–800 mg PO qd Itraconazole‡ 200 mg PO bid		*Meningitis:* Intrathecal amphotericin B usually added for coccidioidomycosis meningitis Fluconazole preferred for meningitis (Ann Intern Med 1993;119:28)
Maintenance	Fluconazole 400 mg/day Itraconazole‡ 200 mg PO bid	Amphotericin B 1 mg/kg/wk	*Drug selection:* Fluconazole often preferred because of more predictable absorption and fewer drug interactions (Antimicrob Agents Chemother 1995;39:1907) *Immune reconstitution:* Maintenance therapy is lifelong regardless of immune reconstitution
Prophylaxis			*Not recommended*
PENICILLIN MARFENII (Penicilliosis)	Amphotericin B 0.7–1.0 mg/kg/day Itraconazole 200 mg PO bid		Fever ± pneumonitis, adenopathy, skin, and mucosal lesions (papules, nodules, or pustules)

			Where: Endemic in Thailand, Hong Kong, China, Vietnam, and Indonesia (Emerg Infect Dis 1996;2:109; Lancet 1994;344:110). Drug select in vitro sensitivity tests show good activity for amphotericin B, ketoconazole, itraconazole, miconazole, and 5FC (J Mycol 1995; Med 5:21; AAC 1993;37:2407)
Maintenance	Itraconazole 200 mg po/d	Ketoconazole	Lifelong treatment required (NEJM 1998; 339:1739)

PARASITIC INFECTIONS

***TOXOPLASMA GONDII* ENCEPHALITIS Acute infection (CID 1996;22:266)**	Pyrimethamine + folinic acid (see preferred regimen) combined with one of the following • Clindamycin 600 mg IV q6h or PO q6h • Atovaquone 150 mg mg bid • Azithromycin 90–1200 mg/d po TMP-SMX 5 mg/kg TMP bid IV or PO Atovaquone 1.5 g bid ± sulfadiazine 1–1.5 gm q6h *Miscellaneous regimens* • Pyrimethamine + leukovorin + clari 500 mg bid • Minocycline doxycycline + pyrimethamine or sulfadiazine or clindamycin	*Response:* Anticipated response is clinical improvement within 1 wk and improvement by CT scan or MRI within 2 wk (CID 2000;30:49) *Failure:* Failure to respond and/or uncertain diagnosis is usually an indication for stereotactic brain biopsy, which has excellent diagnostic yield and good safety record (CID 2000;30:49) Corticosteroids if significant edema/ mass effect (Decadron 4 mg PO or IV q6h) *Trial data:* Controlled trial in 340 patients showed pyrimethamine (50 mg/day) plus sulfadiazine (4 g/day × 8 wk, then 2 g/day) was superior to pyrimethamine (50 mg/day) plus clindamycin (2.4 g/day × 8 wk, then 1.2 g/day) (CID 1996;22:268) *Alternative:* For alternative regimens see TMP-SMX (AAC 1998;42:1346) Atovaquone + sulfa (CID 2002;34: 1243) Pyrimethamine + azithromycin, clarithromycin or clarithromycin (AAC 1991;35:2049) Pyrimethamine + atovaquone (CID 2002;34:1243)

Pyrimethamine 200 mg loading dose, then 50 mg (<60 kg) or 75 mg (>60 kg) mg/day PO + folinic acid 10–20 mg/day PO + sulfadiazine 1 gm (<60 kg) or 1.5 g (>60 kg) × ≥ 6 wk

Table 42. (continued)

	Preferred Regimen(s)	Alternative Regimen(s)	Comments
		PARASITIC INFECTIONS	
T. gondii encephalitis Suppressive therapy	1. Continue half dose pyrimethamine, sulfadiazine clindamycin or TMP-SMX or 2. Pyrimethamine 50 mg qd po + leukovorin 15 mg po/d + sulfadiazine 1 g q1z	Alternatives without established efficacy; Pyrimethamine 25-75 mg/d PO + folinic acid 10-25 mg qd + either atovaquone 750 mg q8-12hr, dapsone* 100 mg/day PO, or azithromycin 600 mg/day PO	*Prophylaxis:* Pyrimethamine-sulfadiazine, TMP-SMX (TDS/d), and atovaquone ± pyrimethamine provide *P. carinii* prophylaxis; pyrimethamine-clindamycin does not *Duration:* Treatment is lifelong unless there is immune reconstitution (see following)
T. gondii encephalitis Prophylaxis (see pg 50)			
CRYPTOSPORIDIUM (Clin Microbiol Rev 1999;12:554; CID 2001;32:331, NEJM 2002;346:1723)	HAART Symptomatic treatment with supplements and antidiarrheal agents: Lomotil, loperamide, paregoric, bismuth subsalicylate (Pepto-Bismol)	Paromomycin 500 mg PO tid or 1000 mg PO bid with food × 14-28 days, then 500 mg PO bid Paromomycin 1 g bid + azithromycin 600 mg qd × 4 wk, then paromomycin alone × 8 wk Azithromycin 1200 mg × 2 PO 1st day, then 1200 mg/day × 27 days, then 600 mg/day, or clarithromycin 500 mg PO bid Atovaquone 750 mg PO suspension with meal bid Nitazoxanide 500 mg PO bid	*Rx:* Trials with paromomycin show inconsistent modest improvement and no cures (Am J Med 1996;100: 370) One reported uncontrolled trial of paromomycin plus azithromycin showed good response in terms of clinical symptoms and oocyst excretion (JID 1998;178:900). Azithromycin alone is ineffective Nitazoxanide (Unimed Pharmaceuticals, Buffalo Grove, IL) is approved for pediatric use. In ACTG 192 about 30% of adults responded. Usual dose is 500 mg PO bid and may be increased to 2000 mg/day HAART with immune reconstitution is most effective treatment (Lancet 1998;351:256, 1998; AIDS 12:35

...inflammatory agents are sometimes useful. Nutritional supplements often required for severe cases; Vivonex TEN or parenteral hyperalimentation
Prophylaxis: Clarithromycin or rifabutin prophylaxis for MAC prophylaxis may reduce risk of cryptosporidiosis (JAMA 1998;279:384)

ISOSPORA **Acute infection** (CID 32:331; 2001; NEJM 1989;320:1044)	Trimethoprim + sulfamethoxazole PO bid (2 DS PO bid or 1 DS tid) × 2-4 wk	Pyrimethamine 50-75 mg/d PO + folinic acid 5-10 mg/day × 1 mo	*Duration:* Duration of high-dose therapy is not well defined *Alternatives:* One case report of refractory infection responded to pyrimethamine plus sulfadiazine (Diagn Microbiol Infect Dis 1996;26:87)
Suppressive treatment	Trimethoprim + sulfamethoxazole 1-2 DS/day or 3×/wk	Pyrimethamine 25 mg + sulfadoxine 500 mg PO q wk (1 Fansidar/wk) Pyrimethamine 25 mg + folinic acid 5 mg/day	*Duration:* Treat indefinitely unless there is immune reconstitution
MICROSPORIDIOSIS (CID 2001;32:331)	HAART Symptomatic treatment with nutritional supplements and antidiarrheal agents (Lomotil, Loperamide, paregoric, etc.) Albendazole 400 mg PO bid × ≥ 3 wk (*E. intestinalis*) Fumagillin 60 mg/day × 14 day (*E. bieneusi*)	Metronidazole 500 mg PO tid Atovaquone 750 mg PO tid with meals bid (AIDS 1996;10:619) Thalidomide 100 mg qd (AIDS 1995; 9:658) Nitazoxanide 500 mg PO bid	*Fumagillin:* Controlled trial showed efficacy of fumagillin for *E. bieneusi* infections, but high rate of thrombocytopenia and neutropenia (NEJM 2002;346:1963) *Albendazole:* Efficacy of albendazole is established only for infections involving *E. intestinalis,* which cause 10-20% of cases *Miscellaneous agents:* Anecdotal success with itraconazole, fluconazole, atovaquone, and metronidazole (Infect Dis Clin North Am 1994;8:483) *HAART:* HAART with immune reconstitution is the best therapy, especially for the 80-90% of cases involving *E. bieneusi* (Lancet 1998;351:256; J AIDS 2000;25:124)

Table 42. (continued) TUBERCULOSIS TREATMENT RECOMMENDATIONS (Statement of the CDC, IDSA and ATS: Am J Resp Crit Care Med 2003;167:603)

Induction	Maintenance*	Comments
RIFAMPIN-BASED THERAPY (NO CONCURRENT USE OF PIs OR NNRTIs with 3 exceptions (see comments)		
1. INH/RIF/PZA/EMB (or SM) daily × 2 mo (preferred if CD4 count <100/mm³)	INH/RIF daily or 2–3×/wk × 18 wk	RIF-containing regimens preclude concurrent use of protease inhibitors and NNRTI other than EFV or SQV/RTV
2. INH/RIF/PZA/EMB (or SM) daily × 2 wk, then 2–3×/wk × 6 wk	INH/RIF or 2–3×/wk × 18 wk	A 2-wk washout is required between last RIF dose and initiation of PI or NNRTIs
3. INH/RIF/PZA/EMB (or SM) 3×/wk × 8 wk	INH/RIF/PZA/EMB (or SM) 3×/wk × 4 mo	
RIFABUTIN-BASED THERAPY (CONCURRENT PI OR NNRTI)		
1. INH/RFB/PZA/EMB daily × 8 wk (preferred if CD4 count <100/mm³)	INH/RFB daily or 2–3×/wk × 18 wk	Dose modifications of RFB and PIs/NNRTI when given concurrently (see Table 38 next page)
2. INH/RFB/PZA/EMB daily × 2 wk, then 2×/wk × 6 wk	INH/Rifabutin 2–3×/wk × 18 wk	

INH, isoniazid; RIF, rifampin; RFB, rifabutin; EMB, ethambutol; PZA, pyrazinamide; SM, streptomycin.

Table 42. (continued)
Directly Observed Therapy Two to Three Times Per Week Preferred
(Statement of CDC, ATS, and IDSA (Am J Resp Crit Care Med 2003;167:603;
http.www.cdc.gov/nchstp/tb/pubs/mmwr/rr4720.pdf)

	Daily	2×/wk	3×/wk
Isoniazid (INH)	5 mg/kg (300 mg)*	15 mg/kg (900 mg)*	15 mg/kg (600 mg)*
Rifampin*** (RIF)	10 mg/kg (600 mg)*	10 mg/kg (600 mg)*	10 mg/kg (600 mg)*
Rifabutin (RFB)	150–450 mg**	300–450 mg**	300–450 mg**
Pyrazinamide (WT) 40–55 kg 56–75 kg ≥75 kg	 1.0 g 1.5 g 2.0 g	 2.0 g 3.0 g 4.0 g	 1.5 g 2.5 g 3.0 g
Ethambutol (WT) 40–55 kg 56–75 kg 76–90 kg	 800 mg 1200 mg 1600 mg	 2000 mg 2800 mg 4000 mg	 3200 mg 2000 mg 2400 mg
Streptomycin (SM)	15 mg/kg (1 g)*	15 mg/kg (1.5 g)*	15 mg/kg (1.5 g)*

* Maximum dose.
** Rifabutin (RFB) to be used with PIs or NNRTIs. See doses below.
*** Rifampin may be used in standard dose with efavirenz, ritonavir, or ritonavir + saquinavir. The SQV/RTV regimens include 400/400 mg bid and 1000/100 mg bid, 1600/100, or
2000/100 mg qd.

TB Treatment Recommendations (continued)
Options for antiretroviral therapy (Am J Resp Crit Care Med 2003;167:603)
  • Regimen that does not contain a PI or NNRTI with exceptions below
  • Streptomycin-based therapy with no use of rifamycins
  • Rifabutin-based treatment with dose adjustments
  • Use rifampin-based regimen with efavirenz, ritonavir, or ritonavir +
    saquinavir (standard doses for both drugs)
Rifabutin regimens (MMWR 2004;53:37)

PI or NNRTI	Rifabutin*
Indinavir 1000 mg q8h	150 mg/day or 300 mg 2–3×/wk
Nelfinavir 1000 mg tid or 1250 mg bid	150 mg/day or 300 mg 2–3×/wk
Amprenavir or Fosamprenavir—Standard dose	150 mg/day or 300 mg 2–3×/wk
Efavirenz 600 mg qd	450 mg/day or 600 mg 2–3×/wk
Nevirapine 200 mg bid	300 mg/day or 300 mg 2–3×/wk
Lopinavir/ritonavir 400/100 mg bid	150 mg qod or 150 mg 2–3×/wk
Ritonavir 600 mg bid	150 mg qod or 150 mg 2–3×/wk
PI boosted with RTV: PI-standard	150 mg qod or 150 mg 3×/wk

Contraindicated: Delavirdine and saquinavir (without RTV).
  * Regimens advocated for 2–3 ×/wk should be 3 ×/wk with CD4 <100/mm^3

Table 42. (continued)

	Preferred Regimen(s)	Alternative Regimen(s)	Comments
TB prophylaxis (see p 49)			
Paradoxical worsening with HAART or immune recovery TB	Antituberculosis drugs + anti-inflammatory drugs		*Features:* Characterized by fever, lymphadenopathy, and pleural effusion usually several weeks after HAART. AFB stains and cultures are often negative (Am J Respir Crit Care Med 1998;158:157; Am J Med 1999;106:371; CID 1998;26: 1008)
MYCOBACTERIUM AVIUM COMPLEX (MAC) BACTEREMIA Treatment	Clarithromycin 500 mg PO bid plus ethambutol 15 mg/kg/day PO. ±Rifabutin 300 mg/d po (severe disease)	Azithromycin 600 mg/day PO + ethambutol ± rifabutin Combination treatment with amikacin 10–15 mg/kg/day IV or ciprofloxacin 500–750 mg bid	*Duration:* Duration is indefinite in absence of immune reconstitution Discontinue maintenance if CD4 count >100/mm³ × 6 mo, ≥12 mo therapy and asymptomatic *Clarithromycin levels:* increased 50–80% with concurrent indinavir, ritonavir, saquinavir and delavirdine, but standard doses are recommended. APVr and NVP have no clinically significant effect. No data for NFV or LPV/r. Avoid EFV *In vitro susceptibility* tests are not useful in previously untreated patients (CID 1998; 27:1369) and are most useful post treatment for clarithromycin

Trials: azithromycin vs clarithromycin for MAC bacteremia showed clarithromycin was superior in time to negative blood cultures (CID 1998;27:1278); another trial showed these macrolides (+ ethambutol) were comparable (CID 2000;31:1254)

Rifabutin dose adjustments: with concurrent PIs or NNRTIs: See p 98,155

Drug interaction between clarithromycin and rifabutin results in 50% decrease in clarithromycin levels and 56% increase in RBT levels (NEJM 335:428, 1996; JID 181: 1289, 2000). Avoid clarithromycin and rifampin

Symptomatic Rx: ASA or NSAID often effective for symptom relief

Clarithromycin at a dose >1000 mg/day was associated with increased mortality (Ann Intern Med 1994;121:905)

MAC prophylaxis: See
p 48

MAC immune recovery lymphadenitis

Continue treatment for MAC and HAART Symptomatic Rx with NSAIDS; if sx severe give prednisone (20–40 mg/day with rapid taper) Surgical drainage of focal lesions often required

Clinical features: Characterized by high-fever leukocytosis and lymphadenopathy, often involving the periaortic and mesenteric nodes. Less common presentations: bursitis, osteomyelitis, skin nodules, adrenal insufficiency. Biopsy shows granulomatous lymphadenitis with AFB in large numbers. Occurs within 1–3 mo of HAART (Lancet 1998;351:252; J AIDS 1999; 20:122; Ann Intern Med 2000;133:447; Clin Infect Dis 2004;38:461)

Table 42. (continued)

	Preferred Regimen(s)	Alternative Regimen(s)	Comments
MYCOBACTERIUM KANSASII	INH 300 mg PO/day + rifampin 600 mg/day PO + ethambutol 15–25 mg/kg/day PO × 18 mo and for at least 15 mo after sputum conversion ± streptomycin 1 g IM 2 × /wk × 3 mo	Also consider ciprofloxacin 750 mg PO bid and clarithromycin 500 mg PO bid	*Experience in HIV-infected patients:* limited (J AIDS 1991;4:516; Ann Intern Med 1991; 114:861) *Duration of therapy is arbitrary* *In vitro activity:* All strains are resistant to PZA
MYCOBACTERIUM HAEMOPHILUM	INH + rifampin + ethambutol	Clarithromycin, doxycycline, ciprofloxacin, and amikacin	*Experience:* limited (Eur J Clin Microbiol Infect Dis 1993;12:114) *Clinical:* Skin
MYCOBACTERIUM GORDONAE	INH + rifampin + clofazimine or clarithromycin	Streptomycin may be useful	*Presentation:* Disseminated infection like MAC (AIDS 1995;9:659) *Most isolates are contaminants* (Dermatology 1993;187:301; AIDS 1992;6:1217; AAC 1992;36:1987)
MYCOBACTERIUM GENEVENSE	Clarithromycin + ethambutol + rifampin	Other possible agents: Ciprofloxacin, PZA	*Rx:* Clarithromycin-containing regimens are most effective (AIDS 7:1357, 1993)
MYCOBACTERIUM XENOPI	INH/rifampin/ ethambutol/ streptomycin		
MYCOBACTERIUM MALMOENSE	Rifampin/rifabutin/ ethambutol/ clarithromycin or azithromycin		*Presentation:* Pulmonary cavity or CNS (CID 1993;16:540; J Clin Microbiol 1996;34:731)

MYCOBACTERIUM CHELONEI	Clarithromycin 500 mg bid × ≥6 mo	Variable activity: Cefoxitin, amikacin, doxycycline, imipenem, tobramycin, erythromycin	*Presentation:* Skin, soft tissue, bone; Need in vitro sensitivity tests
MYCOBACTERIUM FORTUITUM	Amikacin 400 mg IV q12h + cefoxitin 12 g IV/day × 2–4 wk, then oral agents based on in vitro sensitivity tests	Oral agents—clarithromycin, doxycycline, sulfamethoxazole, ciprofloxacin	*Presentation:* Skin, soft tissue, bone, CNS *Treatment:* ≥3 mo—soft tissue; ≥6 mo for bone involvement

VIRUSES

HERPES SIMPLEX (MMWR 2002;51 (RR-6):13) **Initial treatment: mild**	Acyclovir 400 mg PO 3 × /day or famciclovir 250 mg PO tid or valacyclovir 1.0 g PO bid; all given 7–10 day		*Failure to respond:* Give valacyclovir or give acyclovir IV
Severe or refractory	Acyclovir 15 mg/kg IV/day at least 7 day	Foscarnet 40 mg/kg IV q8h or 60 mg/kg q12h × 3 wk Topical trifluridine as 1% ophthalmic solution q8h	*Failure to respond:* give acyclovir 30 mg/kg/day IV and test sensitivity of isolate to acyclovir *Resistant HSV:* IV foscarnet, topical trifluridine, or high-dose IV acyclovir (12–15 mg/kg IV q8h or by continuous infusion). Relapses after treatment of acyclovir-resistant strains often involve acyclovir-sensitive strains *Topical trifluridine solution* (Viroptic 1%); apply after H_2O_2 cleaning and gentle gauze de'bridement; cover with nonabsorbent gauze with bacitracin and polymyxin ointment

Table 42. (continued)

	Preferred Regimen(s)	Alternative Regimen(s)	Comments
HSV—recurrent	Acyclovir 400 mg PO tid or 800 mg PO bid or famciclovir 125 mg PO bid or valacyclovir 1 g PO bid; all given 5–10 day		*Early treatment*: much more effective
HSV—prophylaxis	Acyclovir 400 mg PO bid or famciclovir 250 mg PO bid or valacyclovir 500 mg–1 g PO qd or bid		*Alternative*: treat each episode Patients receiving ganciclovir, foscarnet, or cidofovir do not require acyclovir prophylaxis *Usual indication*: ≥6 recurrences/yr,* but this may be liberalized with HIV due to evidence indicating increased risk of transmission with HSV shedding (JAIDS 2004;34:435)
Pregnancy	Cesarean section (genital lesions at onset of labor)		*Pregnancy issues*: Acyclovir, famciclovir, and valacyclovir safety is not established in pregnancy, but many authorities endorse acyclovir use with severe primary HSV or severe recurrent disease
HSV—visceral	Acyclovir 15–30 mg/kg IV/day at least 10 day	Foscarnet 40 mg/kg IV q8h × ≥10 days Valacyclovir 1.0 g PO tid	

		Comments
HERPES ZOSTER Dermatomal	Famciclovir 500 mg po tid or valacyclovir 1 g po tid × 7–10 days Pain control: Gabapentin, tricyclics, carbamazepine, lidocaine patch, narcotic.	*Steroids*: Some authorities recommend corticosteroids (Ann Intern Med 1996;125: 376); prednisone 60 mg × 7 day, 30 mg day 8–14, 15 mg day 15–21 *Postherpetic neuralgia*: uncommon in persons <55 yr including AIDS patients *Foscarnet*: preferred for acyclovir-resistant cases *Trial*: Comparative trial of acyclovir vs. valacyclovir showed slight advantage to valacyclovir (AAC 1995;39:1546) *Duration*: Treatment can be started as long as new lesions are forming
VZV—disseminated, ophthalmic nerve involvement or visceral	Acyclovir 30–36 mg/kg IV/day at least 7 day	Acyclovir 30 mg/kg/day IV Foscarnet 40 mg/kg IV q8h or 60 mg/kg IV q12h (especially for acyclovir-resistant strains)
VZV—acyclovir-resistant strains	Foscarnet 40 mg/kg IV q8h or 60 mg/kg q12h	Foscarnet 40 mg/kg IV q8h or 60 mg/kg q12h *Duration*: Role of maintenance therapy unclear
VZV—maintenance (see "Comments")	Acyclovir, famciclovir, or valacyclovir PO in previously noted doses	*Resistance to acyclovir*: unusual (J AIDS 1993;7:254; Ann Intern Med 1991;115:9)
Retinal necrosis	CD4 < 100— Ganciclovir + foscarnet CD4 > 100— Acyclovir IV	*Indication*: Frequent recurrences
VZV—prevention	Varicella zoster immune globulin (ZVIG) 5 vials (6.25 mL) within 96 hr of exposure	Acyclovir 800 mg po 5 × /day × 3 wk (Removed from 2002 CDC/IDSA guidelines due to lack of documented efficacy *Indication*: Exposure to chickenpox or shingles plus no history of either and, if available, negative VZV serology. Preventive treatment must be initiated within 96 hr of exposure and preferably within 48 hr

Table 42. (continued)

	Preferred Regimen(s)	Alternative Regimen(s)	Comments
		VIRUSES	
CYTOMEGALOVIRUS RETINITIS **Initial treatment recommendations** (NEJM 2002;346:1119)	Vision-threatening lesion or immune restoration unlikely: Vitrasert q 6 mo + valganciclovir 900 mg PO/day Immune restoration likely: Above (Vitrasert + valganciclovir or systemic therapy only; ganciclovir 5 mg/kg IV bid × 14-21 day foscarnet 90 mg/kg IV bid × 14-21 day or valganciclovir 900 mg PO bid × 14-21 day	Cidofovir 5 mg/kg IV q wk × 2, then 5 mg/kg q 2 wk + probenecid 2 g PO 3 hr before each dose, 1 g PO at 2 and 8 hr after dose	*Rx principle:* Vitrasert should always be combined with systemic therapy (oral ganciclovir or parenteral agent) to prevent systemic CMV disease and protect contralateral eye *Valganciclovir:* Ganciclovir levels with valganciclovir are comparable to those achieved with IV ganciclovir (NEJM 2002; 346:1119) *Foscarnet:* requires infusion pump, long infusion time, saline hydration *Vitrasert:* superior to IV ganciclovir in time to relapse (220 vs. 71 day), but there is increased risk of involvement of the other eye and increased risk of extraocular CMV disease (NEJM 1997;337:83). Any local therapy should be accompanied by systemic anti-CMV therapy
Maintenance	Valganciclovir 900 mg PO qd Foscarnet IV 90-120 mg/kg day Ganciclovir IV 5-6 mg/kg/day IV 5-7 day/ wk or 1000 mg PO tid Cidofovir 5 mg/kg IV every other week Vitrasert q 6 mo	Intravitreous injections of fomivirsen, ganciclovir, foscarnet, or cidofovir + oral ganciclovir (Ophthalmology 1998;105:1404; Ophthalmology 1995;102:533; NEJM 1999;340: 1063)	*Indications:* Maintenance therapy required lifelong for retinitis in patients without immune recovery *Duration:* Treatment of CMV may be discontinued when the CD4 count is >100-150/mm³ for 3-6 mo providing there is concurrence by an ophthalmologist (JAMA 1999;282:1633; CID 1999;28:528; Ophthalmology 1998; 105:1259; JID 1998;177:1080; JID 1998;177: 1182; Am J Ophthalmol 1998;126:817) *Foscarnet maintenance:* dose is arbitrary; one study showed 120 mg/kg/day was superior to 90 mg/kg/day in survival and time to progression (JID 1993;167:1184)

Progression (on maintenance therapy)	Vitrasert if not used initially Increase dose of same agent to induction doses (ganciclovir 10 mg/kg/day or foscarnet 120 mg/kg/day or valganciclovir 900 mg bid) **or** switch to alternative drug (induction doses)	Cidofovir 5 mg/kg (as previously noted) Fomivirsen 330 μg by intravitreal injection day 1 and 15, then monthly Combination treatment with ganciclovir + foscarnet in maintenance doses (JID 1993; 168:144; Am J Ophthalmol 1994; 117:776; Arch Ophthalmol 1996; 114:23)	*Time to relapse:* varies with definition, use of retinal photographs; and treatment as summarized previously. Subsequent relapses occur more rapidly *Drug selection:* ACTG 228 showed no difference between reinduction with the same drug compared with switching to alternative drug. With combination treatment, there was the best outcome for time to progression (4.8 mo vs. 1.6–2.1 mo) and the worst for quality of life (presumably because of time required for infusions) (Arch Ophthalmol 1996;114: 23) *Ganciclovir-resistance:* Resistance rates to ganciclovir <10% at 3 mo, 25–30% at 9 mo (JID 1998;177:770; AAC 1998;42:2240; JID 2001;183:333; Am J Ophthalmol 2001; 132:700) Best clue is relapse or new lesion in contralateral eye (JID 1998;177:770) *Vitrasert failure:* consider IV or intravitreal foscarnet owing to possible ganciclovir resistance
Immune recovery vitritis		Systemic or periocular corticosteroids continue HAART and CMV therapy	*Presentation:* Posterior segment inflammation in patients with inactive CMV retinitis and immune recovery associated with HAART (Arch Ophthalmol 1998;116:169) *Incidence:* highly variable for reasons that are unclear—up to 40% in some series (JAMA 2000;283:653; Ann Intern Med 2000;133:447; JID 1999;179:697) *Differential:* Must exclude other causes of uveitis including TB, syphilis, toxoplasmosis, lymphoma, and drug reactions (Am J Ophthalmol 1998;125: 292)

Table 42. (continued)

	Preferred Regimen(s)	Alternative Regimen(s)	Comments
VIRUSES			
CYTOMEGALOVIRUS EXTRAOCULAR DISEASE Gastrointestinal	Valganciclovir 900 mg PO bid × 14–21 days Ganciclovir 5 mg/kg IV bid × 14–21 days Foscarnet 60 mg/kg q8h or 90 mg/kg IV q12h × 14–21 days	Failure: Ganciclovir + foscarnet Cidofovir + probenecid	*Colitis Rx:* Ganciclovir and foscarnet are equally effective for CMV colitis (Am J Gastroenterol 1993;88:542) *Duration:* Maintenance therapy should be considered, especially after relapse; discontinuation of maintenance should be considered when CD4 count is >100–150/mm³ × 3–6 mo *Valganciclovir:* Published experience valganciclovir treatment for extraocular CMV is nil, but ganciclovir blood levels are comparable with those achieved with IV ganciclovir (NEJM 2002;346:1119) *Dual therapy:* Foscarnet plus ganciclovir are associated with poor quality of life (JID 1993;167:1184)
Neurologic disease	HAART Ganciclovir + foscarnet IV Valganciclovir PO + foscarnet	Cidofovir	*Combination therapy:* ganciclovir + foscarnet is probably optimal, but quality of life is poor and prognosis with any form of therapy (except possibly HAART) is also poor. Median survival in the HAART era is not significantly prolonged (CID 2002;34:103) *Cidofovir:* Experience is nil with neurologic disease *Maintenance therapy:* should be given after induction phase

Pneumonia	HAART Valganciclovir 900 mg PO bid × ≥21 days Ganciclovir 5 mg/kg IV bid ≥21 day Foscarnet 60 mg/kg q8h or 90 mg/kg IV q12h ≥21 day	Cidofovir + probenecid	*Dx*: Minimum diagnostic criteria: 1) Pulmonary infiltrates; 2) detection of CMV with culture antigen or nucleic acid studies of pulmonary secretions; 3) characteristic intracellular inclusions in lung tissue or bronchoalveolar lavage macrophages; and 4) absence of another pulmonary pathogen (Arch Intern Med 1998;158:957) Consider therapy if there is a copathogen that fails to respond to therapy Long-term maintenance therapy is usually unnecessary unless there is relapse or extrapulmonary end-organ disease
PROGRESSIVE MULTIFOCAL LEUKOENCEPHALOPATHY (PML)	HAART		*Trials*: Multiple studies suggest potential utility of HAART, but results are inconsistent (AIDS 1999;13:1881; CID 1999;28:1152; CID 2000:30: 95). Largest series with 57 patients given HAART showed improvement in 26% and development of new lesions in 16% (JID 2000; 182:1077) Median survival after diagnosis averaged 2–4 mo (NEJM 1998;338:1345; CID 2002;34:103)
BACTERIA			
STREPTOCOCCUS PNEUMONIAE **Treatment**	Penicillin, amoxicillin, cefotaxime, ceftriaxone (see "Comments")	Macrolide, vancomycin, levofloxacin, gatifloxacin, moxifloxacin	*Resistance*: Rates of penicillin resistance increased to about 14–16% in 1998 have stayed relatively flat since then (CID 2003;36:963). The rate of resistance to ceftriaxone and cefotaxime is 2–4% and for fluoroquinolones is 0.5–1%

Table 42. (continued)

	Preferred Regimen(s)	Alternative Regimen(s)	Comments
		BACTERIA	
			Rx resistant strains: Strains highly resistant to penicillin should be treated with linezolid, vancomycin, telithromycin or newer quinolones (levofloxacin, moxifloxacin, gatifloxacin). Macrolides show high rates of resistance but TMP-SMX is now considered inadequate for empiric use owing to high rates of resistance
Prevention	CD4 count >200/mm³: Pneumococcal vaccine 0.5 mL SC	None	*Recommendation:* Repeat at 5-yr intervals or at time of immune recovery with CD4 >200 if initial vaccination was performed when CD4 count was <200/mm³ *Efficacy:* There is little evidence that this vaccine prevents pneumococcal infection but it appears to reduce bacteremia
HAEMOPHILUS INFLUENZAE	Cefuroxime	TMP-SMX Cephalosporins, 2nd and 3rd generation Fluoroquinolones	*Treatment:* Traditional therapy usually adequate (CID 2000:30:461) *H. influenzae* vaccine: *H. influenzae* vaccine is not recommended for adults because most infections involve nonencapsulated strains
NOCARDIA ASTEROIDES	Sulfadiazine or trisulfapyridine 3-12 g PO or IV/day to maintain sulfa level at 15-20 µg/mL TMP-SMX 5-15 mg/kg/d (TMP) PO or IV	Minocycline 100 mg PO bid Other suggested regimens: Imipenem + amikacin; sulfonamide + amikacin or minocycline; ceftriaxone + amikacin	*Regimen:* Sulfonamide dose is determined by severity of illness; pulmonary or skin—low dose; CNS, severe or disseminated disease—high dose *Duration* = >6 mo

Organism			Comments
PSEUDOMONAS *AERUGINOSA*	aminoglycoside + antipseudomonal beta-lactam (ticarcillin, piperacillin, mezlocillin, ceftazidime, cefepime), imipenem, or ciprofloxacin	antipseudomonal beta-lactam (ceftazidime or cefoperazone, cefepime), ciprofloxacin, or imipenem/meropenem	susceptibility data. Need for "double coverage" is disputed
RHODOCOCCUS EQUI	Vancomycin 2 g/d IV ± rifampin 600 mg po qd, ciprofloxacin 750 mg po bid or imipenem 0.5 g IV qid × 2–4 wk plus ciprofloxacin, rifampin or rifampin (above doses)	Erythromycin 2–4 g/day IV Clindamycin TMP-SMX	*Maintenance:* Ciprofloxacin 750 mg PO bid may be used for long-term maintenance, but resistance is likely to develop *Miscellaneous:* Also sensitive to rifampin and aminoglycosides; resistant in vitro to penicillins and cephalosporins
BARTONELLA HENSELAE/ QUINTANA (bacillary angiomatosis)	Erythromycin 250–500 mg PO qid × ≥12 wks Doxycycline 100 mg PO bid ≥12 wk	Other macrolides—clarithromycin 500 mg bid, azithromycin 600 mg/d	*Prevention:* Macrolide for MAC prophylaxis is protective *Duration:* Treat at least 3 mo; if there is relapse—treat life-long *In vitro activity:* does not predict response. Antibiotics quickly reduce microbial load, but clinical response is very slow.
SALMONELLA **Acute** (CID 2001;32:331)	Ciprofloxacin 500 mg PO bid × ≥2 wk	Trimethoprim 5–10 mg/kg/day + sulfamethoxazole IV or 1 DS bid × ≥2 wk (preferred if sensitive) Cephalosporins: 3rd generation	*Relapse:* common. Eradication of *Salmonella* has carrier state been demonstrated only for ciprofloxacin *AZT:* active vs. most *Salmonella* strains and may be effective prophylaxis (JID 1999; 179:1553) *Drug selection* requires in vitro susceptibility data especially for ampicillin. Resistance to fluoroquinolones is rare, but reported (NEJM 2001;344:1572) *Source:* Recommendations are based on IDSA guidelines (CID 2001;32:331)

Table 42. (continued)

	Preferred Regimen(s)	Alternative Regimen(s)	Comments
		BACTERIA	
Maintenance	Ciprofloxacin 500 mg PO bid × several mo	Trimethoprim-sulfamethoxazole 5 mg/kg/day, trimethoprim (1 DS PO bid)	*Indications for maintenance therapy, specific regimens, and duration not well-studied or well-defined*
STAPHYLOCOCCUS AUREUS	*Methicillin-sensitive Staphylococcus aureus (MSSA):* Nafcillin, oxacillin, or cefazolin ± gentamicin and/or rifampin Oral agents: Cefalexin dicloxacillin, clindamycin, ciprofloxacin *Methicillin-resistant Staphylococcus aureus (MRSA):* Vancomycin, daptomycin, and linezolid *Community-acquired MRSA:* • Furunculosis: Drainage ± TMP-SMX • Necrotizing pneumonia: Supportive care + ? TMP-SMX, linezolid, clinda-		*Infections:* S. aureus infections that are common in patients with HIV infection—pyomyositis, tricuspid valve endocarditis, multiple soft tissue infections *Antibiotic selection:* Nosocomial MRSA are often resistant to all drugs other than vancomycin, linezolid, and daptomycin *Community-acquired MRSA:* This is a newly recognized strain of S. aureus, which has an unusual virulence factor (Panton Valentine leukocidine) and a unique mechanism of methicillin resistance (mec IV). It is usually sensitive to TMP-SMX clindamycin and gentamicin. The most common presentation is furunculosis, a rare but devastating necrotizing pneumonia

Treponema pallidum
(MMWR 2002:51:
(RR-6))

Primary secondary
syphilis
and early latent (<1
yr): Benzathine
penicillin G 2.4
mil units IM weekly ×
1
(see "Comments")
Latent syphilis:
Benzathine penicillin
G 2.4 mil units IM
weekly × 3
Neurosyphilis: Aqueous
penicillin G 18–24 mil
units/day IV × 10–14
days (3–4 mil units
q4h)

No alternative considered adequate
for HIV-infected patients; If history
of penicillin allergy then perform
skin test if reagents available (major
and minor)—If positive skin test or
positive history and no skin test then
desensitize
Ceftriaxone (CID 2000:30:540)

Follow-up: primary and secondary cases
clinically and serologically at 3, 6, 9, 12 mo
and 24 mo; latent syphilis: serology at 6, 12,
18, and 24 mo
Definition late latent: Patients with latent
syphilis of uncertain duration are considered
to have late latent syphilis
Lumbar puncture: recommended with
neurologic symptoms, treatment failure, and
late latent syphilis

* Patients with G-6-PD deficiency are at risk for hemolytic anemia when given oxidant drugs such as dapsone, sulfonamides, and primaquine. Some advocate screening all potential recipients, some restrict screening to persons at greatest risk (African-American men, men of Mediterranean descent, men from India or Far East); some simply observe for evidence of hemolysis, which usually occurs in first several days of treatment and often resolves with continued administration. Patients with the Mediterranean variant are at risk for severe hemolysis.

Liquid formulation of itraconazole is preferred to capsules for thrush, for patients with achlorhydria, and those with subtherapeutic trough serum levels with capsules (<2 μg/mL); some consider the liquid formulation to be the preferred form for all oral itraconazole therapy, although all clinical trials except for thrush and *Candida* esophagitis were conducted with the capsule form.

Abbreviations:
AMB, amphotericin B

AMP, amprenavir
ATV-atazanavir
AZT, zidovudine
Cipro, ciprofloxacin
CMV, cytomegalovirus
CT, computed
tomographic scan
DLV, delavirdine
EFV, efavirenz
EMB, ethambutol
FPV, fosamprenavir
5-FC, flucytosine
(5-fluorocytosine)
FUO, fever of unknown
origin
G-CSF, granulocyte
colony-stimulating
factor

HAART, highly active
antiretroviral therapy
INH, isoniazid
MRI, magnetic resonance
imaging
NFV, nelfinavir
NVP, nevirapine
Oflox, ofloxacin
PCP, *P. carinii* pneumonia
PZA, pyrazinamide
RBT, rifabutin
Rif, rifampin
RTV, ritonavir
SMX, sulfamethoxazole
SQV, saquinavir
Strep, streptomycin
TMP, trimethoprim

Immune Reconstitution Syndrome: The following summarizes highlights of IRS (CID 2004; 38:1159)

- MAC-associated IRS account for about one third of all reported cases.
- The interval between initiation of ART and the onset of IRS ranges from less than one week to several months, but most occur during the first eight weeks.
- The CD4 count at baseline is usually less than 50 cells/mm^3 at the initiation of ART and then increases at least 2–4 fold during the subsequent 12 months accompanied by a substantial decrease in HIV viral load.
- HIV-specific immunity is generally not adequately reconstituted (*Letvin NL Nat Med 2003;9:861*).
- IRS occurs in two settings: one in which ART is started at the time the patient is undergoing treatment for the OI which accounts for the preference by some physicians to avoid initiation of HAART during this period with infections caused by *P. carinii* or *M. tuberculosis*. The second pattern is when HAART is given to a clinically stable patient.
- The usual treatment consists of symptomatic management using nonsteroidal anti-inflammatory drugs, sometimes with steroids, usually with continued ART and specific treatment directed against the specific pathogen. However, there are individual variations to this and treatment guidelines are often lacking.

Examples of multiple pathogens, the clinical features and management guidelines are summarized in the following table:

Pathogen	Clinical Features	Management
M. avium	Skin, adenitis, pul. infiltrates, liver granuloma mediastinitis, osteo, cerebritis	ART, Antibiotics ± steroids
M. tuberculosis	Pneumonitis, ARDS, adenitis, hepatitis, CNS TB, renal failure, epididymitis	ART, Antibiotics ± steroids
M. leprae	Cutaneous lesion	ART, dapsone
Cryptococcosis	Meningitis, palsy, hearing loss, abscess, mediastinitis, adenitis	ART, Azole, steroids
P. carinii	Pneumonia	ART, Antibiotics, steroids
HBV & HCV	Hepatitis	ART ? D/C, TDF ± 3TC
JC virus	CNS lesions, inflammation	ART, steroids, cidofovir
BK virus	Hemorrhagic cystitis	ART, symptomatic therapy
HSV	Chronic erosive ulcers, encephalitis	ART, antivirals, steroids
VZV	Zoster flare	ART, antivirals, steroids
CMV	Vitritis, cytoid macular edema, uveitis, vitreomacular traction	ART, IVIG, steroids, vitrectomy, antivirals
KS	Tracheal mucosal edema, obstruction	D/C ART, steroids
HPV	Inflamed warts, mollusca contagiosa	Steroids, surgery
Parvovirus B19	Focal encephalitis	D/C ART, IVIG
HIV	Demyelinating leukoencephalopathy	D/C ART, steroids
C. trachomatis	Reiter syndrome, urethritis, arthritis	Doxycycline

Table 43. Treatment of Miscellaneous and Noninfectious Disease Complications Classified by Organ System

Condition	Treatment	Comments
Cardiac Cardiomyopathy J AIDS 1998;18:145; (NEJM 1998;339:1153; Am J Cardiol 1999;83: 1A)	ACE inhibitors, (i.e., enalapril 2.5 mg bid titrated to 20 mg/day as tolerated or captopril 6.25 mg tid titrated to 50 mg tid or lisinopril 10 mg/day titrated to 40 mg/d Failure to respond: add diuretic hydrochlorothiazide 25–50 mg/day furosemide 10–40 mg/day, or spironolactone 25–100 mg/day Refractory: Add digoxin 0.125–0.25 mg/day HAART	*Dx:* Echocardiograms show dilated cardiomyopathy in up to 8% of HIV-infected patients (NEJM 1998;339:1093). *Sx:* Subclinical cardiac abnormalities are common and correlate with extent of immune suppression (BMJ 1994;309:1605; NEJM 1998;339:1153) *ID causes:* Infectious causes: are: *T. gondii,* TB, *C. neoformans,* CMV
Pulmonary Lymphoid interstitial pneumonitis or non-specific interstitial pneumonitis	HAART Prednisone dose unclear	*Etiology:* Possibly caused by HIV infection of the lung *Sx:* Clinical presentation and x-ray resemble PCP, but CD4 is often 200–500. Some patients respond when inadvertently treated for PCP (Am J Respir Crit Care Med 1997;156:912) *Steroids:* Indications and optimal dose of corticosteroid treatment not established; most initiate this treatment after initial observation shows progression; maintenance prednisone sometimes required
Pulmonary hypertension	Diuretics Epoprosterol Sildenafil 25 mg/day titrate up to 25 mg tid (AIDS 2001;15:1747; NEJM 2000;343:1342)	*HHV-8:* may be cause (NEJM 2003;349: 1113) Role of HHV-8 antiviral therapy (ganciclovir, foscarnet, or cidofovir). *Dx:* Doppler echo or cardiac cath

Renal
Nephropathy (HIV-associated nephropathy—HIVAN)

Antiretroviral therapy (HAART) (Lancet 1998: 352:783; NEJM 2001;344:1979)

Hemodialysis (Am J Kidney Dis 1997;29:549)

Hemodialysis and peritoneal dialysis appear equally effective (Am J Kidney Dis 1990;16:1)

Prednisone 60 mg/day × 2–11 wk, then taper 10 mg/wk × 2–26 wk (Am J Med 1994;97:145; Kidney Internat 2000;58:1253)

ACE inhibitors: Captopril 6.25–25 mg PO tid or other inhibitors (J Ped 119:710, 1991; J Am Soc Nephrol 8:1140, 1997): Results are variable

Transplantation: Preliminary results in 23 patients with response to HAART and CD4 > 200 showed graft survival in 87% (Kid Internat 2003;63:1618)

Most common form is collapsing focal glomerulosclerosis; onset with nephrosis and rapid course to end-stage renal disease in 1–4 mo (Kidney Int 1995;48: 311)

Must distinguish from renal disease due to 1) heroin-associated acute tubular necrosis, 2) renal failure due to drugs including indinavir and tenofovir, 3) renal failure due to common predisposing conditions such as diabetes and HBP, and 4) immune complex nephritis due to HCV mixed cryoglobulinemia (Ann Intern O Med 2003;139:214). Features of HIVAN are heavy proteinuria, rapid progression, absence of edema, absence of hypertension, and normal-sized kidneys

Risks for HIVAN are African-American race, CD4 count <200/mm^3, lack of ART (AIDS 2004;18:541)

Response to steroids is variable and temporary; regimen in ACTG 271 was prednisone 60 mg/day × 6 wk, then taper 10 mg/wk × 6 wk. Uncontrolled trial of 60 mg/day × 2–11 wk with taper over 2–26 wk showed decrease in creatinine in 17/19 and decreased proteinuria in 12/13 (Am J Med 1996;101: 41); five relapsed and responded to retreatment

Response to HAART based on clinical and biopsy data has been reported (Lancet 1998;352:783; Clin Nephrol 2002;57:335; NEJM 2001;344:1979)

Table 43. (continued)

Condition	Treatment	Comments
Neurologic Peripheral neuropathy	Discontinue implicated NRTIs (ddC, d4T, ddl) Lamotrigine (Lamactal) 25 mg PO bid increasing to 300 mg/day over 6 wk Nortriptyline 10 mg hs: Increase dose by 10 mg q 5 day to maximum of 75 mg hs or 10-20 mg PO tid Ibuprofen 600-800 mg tid Topical: Capsaicin-containing ointments (Zostrix, etc). Lidocaine 20-30% ointment for topical use Alternatives: Phenytoin 200-400 mg/day and carbamazepine 200-400 mg PO bid Neurontin (gabapentin): 300-1200 mg PO tid	Tricyclics commonly used include nortriptyline, amitriptyline, desipramine, or imipramine—efficacy not established (JAMA 1998;282:1590) Lamotrigine is only drug with significant benefit vs. placebo in a controlled trial (Neurology 54:2115) Capsaicin is usually not well tolerated Mexiletine appeared no better than placebo and was inferior to amitriptyline in ACTG 242 One report of two patients suggests response to HAART (Lancet 1998;352:1906) Acupuncture: A controlled trial failed to show any benefit (JAMA 1998;280:1590) Nucleosides that cause peripheral neuropathy are ddC, ddl and d4T. Rank order: ddl/d4T > d4T > ddl (AIDS 2000;14: 273)
Acute neuropathy and lactic acidosis	Discontinue NRTIs	Described in 2002; 25 cases reported to FDA Cause: NRTI-induced mitochondrial toxicity, especially d4T (NEJM 2002;346:811) Clinical definition: Ascending paresis, areflexia and cranial neuropathies. Laboratory tests show elevated lactate and CPK may be acute (1-2 wk) or subacute (>2 wk)

HIV-associated dementia (HAD)	Possible benefit from antiretroviral regimens with agents that penetrate CNS (AZT, d4T, ABC, IDV, NVP), less but good penetration—EFV, ddI, 3TC, and APV (AIDS 1998;12:537; JAIDS 1998;235:238) Anecdotal experience indicates response to HAART	Benefit of AZT at higher dose for mild or moderately severe HAD is established Monitor therapy with neurocognitive tests such as HIV Dementia Scale (AIDS Reader 2002;12:29) CSF levels of HIV RNA respond to HAART in some but not all; response correlates with baseline CD4 count and plasma HIV RNA levels HAART: Response with immune reconstitution is variable, but the changes appear less impressive than with other HIV-associated complications (AIDS 1999;13:1249; AIDS 2001;15:195; J Neurovirol 2002;8:136)
Hematologic *Idiopathic thrombocytopenic purpura (ITP)* Asymptomatic	HAART Discontinue any drugs potentially responsible: Rifampin, amphotericin, ethambutol, sulfas, lithium	Note: Standard treatments (prednisone, IVIG, splenectomy, etc) show response rates of 40–90%; main problem is lack of a durable response (CID 1995;21:415) Response to AZT may be dose-related; usually responds within 2–4 wk. Utility of other nucleoside analogs is unknown Average increase in platelet count with HAART is 18,000–45,000 at 3 mo (CID 2000;30:504; NEJM 1999;341:1239)
Severe hemorrhage	Packed red cell/platelet transfusions **plus** prednisone 60–100 mg/day or IVIG 1 g/kg on day 1, 2, 14, and then q 2–3 wk	

Table 43. (continued)

Condition	Treatment	Comments
Persistent symptomatic ITP	Discontinue implicated drugs and avoid nonsteroidal antiinflammatory drugs. HAART	Initial results with HAART show good response (NEJM 1999;341:1239)
	Prednisone 30–60 mg/day with rapid taper to 5–10 mg/day	Prednisone may be complicated by opportunistic infections, especially thrush and herpes and decreased CD4 count; only 10–20% have persistent response
	IVIG 400 mg/kg day 1, 2, 14, and then q2–3wk or	IVIG is highly effective in raising platelet count within 4 day but is expensive, and median duration of response is only 3 wk
	WinRho 25–50 μg/kg IV over 3–5 min, repeat at day 3–4 pm; may need maintenance therapy at 3- to 4-wk intervals using 25–60 μg/kg	WinRho is an alternative to IVIG in Rh-positive ITP patients. Advantages are 3- to 5-min infusions, good safety profile, and reduced cost (Blood 1991;77:1884)
	Splenectomy	Utility with splenectomy is debated: durability of response is variable and some claim risk of HIV progression is increased (Lancet 1987;2:342); others claim good long-term results (Arch Surg 1989;124:625)
	Splenic irradiation, danazol, vincristine, interferon	Experimental or experience limited with all four

Anemia

Treatment based on cause
HAART

Three causes are 1) decreased production: infiltration tumor (lymphoma, KS), infection (MAC, TB, parvovirus B 19, CMV, histoplasmosis), drugs (AZT, amphotericin, ganciclovir, hydroxyuria, phenytoin, TMP-SMX, ribavirin, pyrimethamine, interferon), anemia of chronic disease, deficiency state (Fe, vitamin B$_{12}$, folic acid) or HIV inhibition of precursors (CID 2000:30:405); 2) increased destruction (hemolysis) TTP, drugs (sulfonamides, dapsone, primethamine + G6PD deficiency); 3) blood loss

Parvovirus B 19: IVIG 400 mg/kg/day × 5 day (Ann Intern Med 1990;113:926)

Parvovirus B 19: Marrow shows giant pronormoblasts with clumped basophilic chromatin and clear cytoplasmic vacuoles—diagnosis by in situ hybridization to show virus

Anemia algorithm for EPO
EPO candidate: Hct <30%, Hgb <9 g/dL

Exclude bleeding (stool guaiac), hemolysis (smear), and iron deficiency (serum iron, transferrin, % saturation, and ferritin)

↓
Underlying cause
↓
Correct
↓
Initiate EPO 40,000 units SC q wk (± supplemental iron)

Monitor response that will usually not be seen for ≥2 wk

Hgb ↑ >1 g/dL at 4 wk: Continue same dose   Hgb increase <1 g/dL at 4 wk: Increase to 60,000 units q wk

Monitor therapy at this dose

Hgb >11-13 g/dL: Hold EPO or decrease by 10,000 units/wk   Hgb increase <1 g/dL at wk 12: Discontinue

Table 43. (continued)

Condition	Treatment	Comments
Neutropenia	Discontinue drugs that cause neutropenia when possible HAART	Most likely agents: AZT, ganciclovir and valganciclovir; others, ddI, d4T, foscarnet, ribavirin, flucytosine, amphotericin, pentamidine, pyrimethamine, sulfonamide antineoplastic agent, and interferon
	G-CSF (Neupogen) or GM-CSF (Leukine) 1–10 µg/kg/day SC; usual initial dose of G-CSF is 5 µg/kg/day with increases of 1 µg/kg/day at 5- to 7-day intervals to maintain ANC at 1000–2000/mm³; usual maintenance dose is 300 µg given 3–7×/wk (NEJM 1987;371:593)	Reported risk of neutropenia is variable; largest analysis showed higher risk for hospitalization with ANC <500 (Arch Intern Med 1997;157:1825); but results are variable (CID 2001;32:469) G-CSF therapy. Monitor with CBC and differential 2×/wk and titrate up by 1 µg/kg/day or reduce dose 50% q wk for maintenance to keep ANC >1000–2000/mL. Efficacy of G-CSF is established for AIDS patients (NEJM 1987;317:593) HAART: Response with immune reconstitution is variable (CID 2000;30:504; J AIDS 2001;28:221)
Thrombotic thrombocytopenic purpura	Prednisone 60–100 mg/day plus plasmapheresis (NEJM 1991;325:393)	Average of 7–16 exchanges required to induce remission

Tumors

Kaposi's sarcoma

ACTG classification (Mayo Clin Proc 1995;70:869)

Good prognosis:
Lesions confined to skin and/or nodes; CD4 >150, no "B symptoms"

Poor prognosis:
Lesion associated edema, severe oral KS, visceral KS, CD4 <150, history of opportunistic infection, or "B symptoms"

Treatment	Comment
General: HAART	KS generally responds to HAART. CD4 count response is best predictor (AIDS 14:971, 987, 2000)
Local therapy Topical liquid nitrogen	Restrict to few lesions that are small
Intralesional vinblastine (0.01–0.002 mg/lesion) q 2 wk × 3	Restrict to few lesions that may be larger (>1 cm)
Radiation (low dose, e.g., 400 rads q wk × 6 wk)	Skin—well tolerated; oral lesion—mucositis common
Laser, cryotherapy	Best with localized lesions Laser, radiation, or vinblastine injection preferred for oral lesions
Systemic therapy	Usually preferred with extensive skin lesions (>25), extensive skin Kaposi's sarcoma (KS) that fails local therapy, visceral involvement (Lancet 1995;346:26)
Liposomal daunorubicin (DaunoXome) 40 mg/m² IV q 2 wk or pegylated liposomal doxorubicin (Doxil) 20 mg/m² IV q 2 wk	Preferred over conventional chemotherapy owing to better response and better tolerance (J Clin Oncol 1998;16:683; J Clin Oncol 1998;16:2445)
Paclitaxel (Taxol)	FDA-approved for KS Considered second line to anthracyclines owing to greater toxicity (marrow suppression) (J Clin Oncol 1998;16:1112). Lower doses (100 mg/m² q 2 wk) preserves efficacy with less toxicity (Cancer 2002;95:147)
Conventional chemotherapy Combinations of adriamycin, bleomycin + vincristine or vinblastin (ABV), bleomycin + vinca alkaloids, or vincristine/vinblastine (alone)	Anthracyclines or paclitaxel are usually preferred (AIDS 1996;10:515)

Table 43. (continued)

Condition	Treatment	Comments
Non-Hodgkin's lymphoma (NHL)	Preferred: M-BACOD (methotrexate, bleomycin, adriamycin, cyclophosphamide, vincristine, and dexamethasone + G-CSF Alternative: EPOCH (etoposide, prednisone, vincristine, cyclophosphamide, and doxorubicin	M-BACOD preferred (NEJM 1997;336:16) Pre HAART results showed good initial response, but short survival (<1 yr) owing to progression of lymphoma or AIDS (Semin Oncol 1998;25:492) Prognosis with chemotherapy + HAART is much better (AIDS 2001;15:1483)
CNS lymphoma	CNS lymphoma—cranial radiation + corticosteroids ± chemotherapy Methotrexate	Standard is radiation + decadron but outcome is poor without HAART (J. Neuro Sci 1999;163:22; Semin Oncol 1998;25;492)
Dermatologic complications		
Bacillary angiomatosis (see pg 167)		
Molluscum contagiosum	Cidofovir—topical Cryotherapy, electrosurgery, curettage, topical cantharidin or cidofovir HAART	Cidofovir is effective when given IV or topically (Lancet 1999;353;2042)
Eosinophilic folliculitis (Internat J Dermatol 1999;37:401)	Permethrin cream + topical high-potency steroids under occlusive dressing Ultraviolet light Antihistamines for pruritis	Dx: Follicular papules and pustules on face, extremities, and trunk; usually very pruritic; CD4 count is usually <250/mm³. Dermpath shows follicular destruction, abscesses, and many eosinophils. Efficacy of UV light established (NEJM 1988; 318:1183) Main complaint is pruritis—need high dose, mixed-class antihistamine (Arch Derm 1995; 131:360) Must distinguish infectious cause—usually S.

Staphylococcal folliculitis	Cephalexin or dicloxacillin 500 mg PO qid × 7–21 day	Add rifampin 600 mg/day × 7 day if severe or refractory Recurrent disease: Chronic antibiotic (clindamycin 150 mg qd or TMP-SMX 1 DS qd) and/or nasal mupirocin
Dermatophytic fungi	Skin (Tinea corporis, T. cruris, T. pedis): Topical agent × 2 wk (T. cruris) to 4 wk (T. pedis) Agents: Clotrimazole (Lotrimin) 1% cream or lotion bid; ecmazole (Spectazole) 1% cream qd or bid, Ketoconazole (Nizoral) 2% cream qd; Terbinafine (Lamisil) 1% cream or gel qd or bid; tolnaftate (Tinactin) 1% cream, gel, powder, solution, acrosol Nails: Itraconazole "pulse therapy" 400 mg/day × 1 wk/mo × 2 mo (fingernails) or 3 mo (toenails) or terbinafine 250 mg/day × 8 wk (fingernails) or 12 wk (toenails)	Topical agents available over the counter: Lotrimin, Lamisil, Monostat—Derm, Tinactin Main concerns with itraconazole: risks of hepatotoxicity, cardiotoxicity and cost Main concerns with terbinafine are risks with treatment of benign condition with drugs that are hepatotoxic and expensive
Seborrhea	Skin—steroid cream (moderate potency—triamcinolone 0.1% or hydrocortisone 2.5%) and/or topical ketoconazole 2% cream applied bid for duration of flare Scalp—shampoos containing selenium sulfide (Selsen, Exelderm), zinc pyrithione (Head and Shoulders, Zincon, DHS zinc), ketoconazole, salicylic acid, or coal tar	Dx: Erythematous plaques with greasy scales—postauricular, presternal, axilla, central face and pubic area. Cause: The yeast Pityrosporum is found in lesions, but may not be the cause in AIDS patients (J Amer Acad Dermatol 1992;27:37)
Gastrointestinal Anorexia	Megace 400–800 mg qd	Weight gain is mostly fat. May lower testosterone levels leading to muscle wasting and impotency consider megace + testosterone
	Dronabinol (Marinol) 2.5 mg PO bid	Synthetic THC is active ingredient in marijuana. Weight gain is mostly fat

Table 43. (continued)

Condition	Treatment	Comments
Nausea/vomiting	Compazine 5–10 mg PO q6–8h; Tigan 250 mg PO q6–8h; Dramamine 50 mg PO q6–8h; Ativan 0.025–0.05 mg/kg IV or IM; haloperidol 1–5 mg bid PO or IM; ondansetron (Zofran) 0.2 mg/kg IV or IM; dronabinol 2.5 mg PO bid	Phenothiazines (Compazine, etc), haloperidol (Haldol), trimethobenzamide (Tigan), and metoclopramide (Reglan) may cause dystonia Must consider medications as cause of nausea Zofran efficacy is established only for cancer chemotherapy and cost is very high
Pancreatitis	Discontinue any implicated drug NPO ± parenteral hyperalimentation Pain control	May be due to adverse drug reaction (especially ddI, d4T, or both, and less frequently: 3TC (?), RTV, LPV/r, INH, rifampin, TMP-SMX, erythromycin, paromomycin, sulfonamides pentamidine) Other causes are EtOH, hyperlipidemia (triglycerides >1000 mg/dL) biliary stone, ERCP, primary HIV infection, or opportunistic infection (CMV, mycobacteria, cryptococcosis) (Am J Med 1995;3:243)
Mouth Aphthous ulcers	Topical treatment: Triamcinalone in orobase Lidex 0.05% ointment in orobase mixed 1:1 Amlexanox 5% oral paste Lidocaine soln before meals Systemic: Prednisone 40 mg/day × 1–2 wk then taper	Classified as minor (<1 cm diameter, usually self limiting in 10–14 day) or major (>1 cm diameter, deep, very painful, may prevent oral intake (AIDS 1992;6: 963) Thalidomide has strict requirements for use but results are good (NEJM 1997;337: 1086)

Condition	Treatment	Comments
	Colchicine 1.5 mg/day Dapsone 100 mg/day Pentoxifylline (Trental) 400 mg PO tid Thalidomide 200 mg/day × 4-6 wk ± maintenance with 200 mg 2× /wk Intralesional steroid	Most treated with antivirals relapse when agent is stopped and may require maintenance therapy Famciclovir, valacyclovir, foscarnet, ganciclovir, valganciclovir should be as effective as acyclovir but have not been studied Most lesions are asymptomatic and do not require treatment
Oral hairy leukoplakia	Usually not treated (except with HAART) Acyclovir 800 mg PO 5× /day × 2-3 wk (Valacyclovir, ganciclovir, foscarnet, valganciclovir, cidofovir should also be effective) Topical podophyllin Cryotherapy	
Salivary gland enlargement	Xerostomia: Sugarless gum and artificial saliva; pilocarpine for refractory cases Painful cystic lesions: Needle aspiration	CT scan distinguishes cystic and solid lesions (Laryngoscope 1988;98:772). Biopsy if malignancy is suspected (most are benign cystic lesions.) Fine-needle aspirate permits microbiologic analysis and decompression
Gingivitis/periodontitis	Curettage and débridement of involved tissue + topical antiseptic such as povidone—iodine solution and chlorhexidine (Peridex) mouth rinses Metronidazole 250 mg tid or 500 mg PO bid × 7-14 days or clindamycin 300 mg PO tid × 7-14 days in selected cases	Four phases: Gingival erythema, necrotizing gingivitis, necrotizing periodontitis, and necrotizing stomatitis (Ann Intern Med 1996;125:485) Usual presenting complaints are oral pain and bleeding
Esophagitis Candida (see p 145)		
Cytomegalovirus (see p 162)		

Table 43. (continued)

Condition	Treatment	Comments
Herpes simplex (see p 159)		
Aphthous ulcer	Prednisone 40 mg/day PO × 2 wk, then slow taper	Need endoscopy and biopsy to exclude microbial cause
	Thalidomide 100–200 mg/day, increase to 400–600 prn as tolerated. When needed D/C thalidomide or use maintenance dose of 50 mg/day	Thalidomide is available through the STEPS program (888-423-5436). Concern is teratogenic side effect. Data for response of aphthous ulcers are good (BMJ 1989;289:432; NEJM 1997;337:1086; AIDS Res Hum Retroviruses 1997;13:301; CID 1995;20:250)
Diarrhea Specific microbial agent CID 2001;32:331	*C. difficile:* Metronidazole 500 mg PO tid × 10–14 day Travelers diarrhea: Ciprofloxacin 500 mg bid × 3 day or TMP-SMX 1 DS bid × 3 day *C. jejuni:* erythromycin 500 mg PO bid × 5 day *Salmonella:* Cipro 500 mg bid × ≥14 day; cefotaxime 4–8 g/d IV × ≥14 day TMP-SMX 1 DS bid × 3 day *Shigella:* Cipro 500 mg bid × 3 day, TMP-SMX 1 DS bid × 3 day *Aeromonas:* TMP-SMX 1 DS bid × 3 day; ciprofloxacin 500 mg bid × 3 day *E. histolytica:* Metronidazole 750 mg PO or IV tid × 5–10 day followed by paromomycin 500 mg PO tid × 7 day Cyclospora: TMP-SMX: DS bid × 3 day	Recommendations are IDSA guidelines (CID 2001;32:331) Antibiotic treatment is contraindicated for diarrhea caused by *E. coli* 0157:H7 (bloody diarrhea without fever) Fluoroquinolone resistance is rare for bacterial pathogens other than *C. jejuni* Many cases are caused by untreatable viruses (NEJM 1993;329:14)

Symptomatic treatment	*Giardia:* Metronidazole 250 mg PO tid CMV (see p 164) MAC (see p 156) × 7–10 day *Cryptosporidia, Isospora,* microsporidia (see p 152)	
	Lomotil/loperamide/paregoric, etc. Diet modification—low fat, no caffeine, no milk, or milk products ± gluten-free diet	Utility of bismuth salts (Pepto-Bismol) and indomethacin unknown Antiperistaltics (Lomotil, loperamide, and narcotics) are contraindicated with *E. coli* 0157:H7 and *C. difficile*
Protease inhibitor associated diarrhea (CID 2000;30:908)	Loperamide—4 mg, then 2 mg with each loose stool, up to 16/day Psyllium 1 tsp bid or 2 bars qd - bid Oat bran 1500 mg bid Calcium 500 mg bid Fiber supplements Pancreatic supplements, 1–2 tabs with meals	Over-the-counter loperamide, psyllium, oat bran, calcium Most common with nelfinavir, loperamide, Fortovase, amprenavir, and ddI

Cholangiopathy

Papillary stenosis	ERCP with sphincterotomy	Presentation: RUQ pain, LFTs show cholestasis; diagnosis established with ERCP. Sensitivity of ultrasound scan is 75–95%
Cholangiopathy without papillary stenosis	Ursodeoxycholic acid 300 mg PO tid (experience limited)	Usual causes are *Cryptosporidium* (most common), microsporidia, CMV, and cyclospora. About 20–40% are idiopathic Treatment directed against microbial pathogen is usually unsuccessful for cholangitis except for cases involving CMV
Isolated duct structure	Endoscopic stenting	Improvement with ursodeoxycholic acid is reported in a small number of patients (Am J Med 1997;103:70)

Table 43. (continued)

Condition	Treatment	Comments
Hepatitis C-HIV co-infection (NIH Consensus Guidelines: Evidence Report #60 AHRQ Pub #02, E030, 7/02 and trials presented at 11th CROI	Hepatitis A vaccine if HAV seronegative Hepatitis B vaccine if susceptible Abstain from or limit alcohol use *Indications for anti-HCV treatment* • HCV RNA >50 IU/mL • Liver biopsy showing portal or bridging fibrosis • No contraindications • Stable HIV preferably with CD4 count >200 **Interferon therapy** Genotype 1: Pegylated interferon plus ribavirin × 48 wk* Genotype 2 and 3: Pegylated interferon plus ribavirin × 48 wk* *Consider discontinuation at 12 wk HCV RNA has not decreased ≥2 log 10 IU/mL *Usual Peg INF-alfa-2a is 180 ug SC/wk plus ribavirin 800 mg/day	*Diagnostic evaluation:* see pp 22 and 35 *Recommendations* based on 3 trials presented at 11th CROI (abstracts 110, 111, 117 B) Results of clinical trials show cure rates of 15-30% with genotype 1 and 60-70% with genotypes 2 and 3 All antiretroviral drugs are potentially hepatotoxic, but chronic HCV infection does not clearly increase risk of hepatotoxicity (JAMA 2000;283:74). Ritonavir and nevirapine are probably the most hepatotoxic Ribavirin can be used with HIV infection, but rate of anemia is high (CID 2000:31: 161) and risk of lactic acidosis due to NRTI-induced mitochondrial toxicity is increased, especially with ddI (Lancet 2001:72:177) Factors that promote progression of HCV-associated liver disease are HIV co-infection and EtOH abuse
Hepatitis B-HIV co-infection (Hepatology 2001;34:1225)	Limit or avoid alcohol use Hepatitis A vaccine if susceptible *Indications to treat* • Evidence of HBV replication: HBeAg + or HBV DNA level >100,000 c/mL *and* • ALT 2x ULN and/or liver bx with necroinflammation	Lamivudine: Early response but rate of resistance by YMDD mutation is 50% at 2 years Tenofovir: Active vs 3TC-resistant HBV; rate of resistance <2% at 1 yr; average decrease in HBV DNA is 4 logs (NEJM 2003;348:177)

	Need to treat HIV but not HBV: Should withhold 3TC and FTC to avoid HBV resistance; consider withholding TDF for same reason *Need to treat both:* Use 3TC + TDF or TDF *Need to treat HBV and not HIV:* Adofovir or interferon	Emtricitabine: Similar to 3TC but experience is limited *Warning:* Discontinuation of 3TC, FTC or TDF may cause HBV flare Adefovir: Active vs 3TC resistant strains; does not appear to promote TDF resistance by HIV. HBV resistance <3% at 3 yr; optimal way to treat HBV without HIV therapy Pegylated interferon: Limited experience with pegylated formulation for HBV; also active vs. HIV
Wasting (NEJM 1999;340:1740)	*Enteral feedings* Polymeric formulas: Ensure, Sustecal, Enrich, Megnacal, etc.	Polymeric formulas: Nonprescription about $1.50/can; 10 cans/day required for total caloric needs. Usually not effective in wasting
	Elemental formulas: Vivonex TEN	Elemental diet for severe malabsorption states; often owing to *Cryptosporidium*, microsporidia, or severe CMV infection; parenteral hyperalimentation and feeding gastrostomy rarely used even in pre-HAART era Parenteral hyperalimentation: Rarely indicated except for devastating diarrhea owing to cryptosporidiosis
	Growth hormone (Serostim) 6 mg SC qd × 12 wk	Most weight gain is lean body mass (Ann Intern Med 1996;125:873) and reduced visceral fat (JAIDS 2002;30:379) Disadvantages are high cost ($1750/wk) need for maintenance therapy and side effects: arthralgias, diabetes, and poor quality of life (JAIDS 2002;30:379)

Table 43. (continued)

Condition	Treatment	Comments
Cytokine suppression	Thalidomide (Thalomid) 50–300 mg/day × 2–12 wk. usual starting dose is 100 mg/day with increase to 200 mg/day if needed	Thalidomide is available through the STEPS program designed to ensure that the men or women do not risk teratogenicity. Call 888-423-5436. Therapeutic trials show good response with weight gain, but high rate of sedation as a side effect (AIDS 1996;10:1501). Not FDA-approved for this use
Appetite stimulants	Megace 400–800 mg/day	Indicated only if weight loss is due to anorexia
	Dronabinol (Marinol) 2.5 mg PO bid	Megace: Weight gain is mostly fat. May lower testosterone levels with impotence; may cause adrenal insufficiency or diabetes (Ann Intern Med 1994;121:400) Dronabinol: Weight gain is limited and mostly fat
Anabolic steroids	Nandrolone 100–200 mg IM q 1–2 wk	Testosterone is preferred when there is documented hypogonadism
	Oxandrolone 20–40 mg/day PO (males). 5–20 mg/day PO (females)	High anabolic effect and low androgenic effect. Most weight gain is lean body mass (AIDS 1996;10:1657) Main concern is hepatic toxicity; Peliosis hepatis, cholestatic hepatitis, and hepatic tumors; other side effects are changes in libido, depression, GI intolerance Safety of nandrolone in women is established by experience with treatment of postmenopausal osteoporosis; main concerns are virilization and teratogenicity with category × rating

Wasting (continued)

Testosterone

Transdermal products

Andro Gel 5 g packet

Androderm 5 mg/day

Testoderm TTS patch 5 mg/day

Parenteral testosterone

Testosterone enanthate or testosterone cypionate 200–400 mg IM q 2 wk or 100–200 mg IM q wk by self-injection

Oxandrolone shows highest weight gain of all treatments

May reverse fat redistribution seen with protease inhibitors

About 50% of men with AIDS in pre-HAART era had hypogonadism; benefit is greatest in this group (NEJM 1999;340: 1740)

Testosterone is available for oral, injectable, or transdermal use. Oral compounds have been associated with liver toxicity; IM injections consist of an ester in oil that extends half-life to permit weekly or biweekly administration. Transdermal patch is changed daily and worn 22 hr/day. Androderm gel permits graduated changes in dose (Med Lett 2000;42:51)

Serum testosterone levels <450 ng/dL are associated with decreased libido. Drugs associated with decreased testosterone levels are megesterol, ketoconazole, and cimetidine

Women with wasting may be treated with testosterone patch according to a placebo-controlled trial with a 4.1 mg patch given 2x/wk (Arch Intern Med 2004;164:897)

Testosterone formulations have high androgenic and anabolic effect with improved mood; increased libido, energy, appetite, and lean body mass (CID 1999;28:634)

Table 43. (continued)

Condition	Treatment	Comments
	Exercise 20 min bicycle or treadmill, then 1 hr resistance training 3×/wk	May be as effective as growth hormone for fat redistribution with HAART (AIDS 1999;13:1373)
	Resistance exercise: 20 min/day × 3 days/wk	Effective in increasing lean body mass; preliminary results suggest efficacy in fat redistribution syndrome ascribed to protease inhibitors
Pain (Med Lett 1993;35:1-6)	ASA, acetaminophen, 325-650 mg q4h	Severe pain is best relieved with opioids
	Nosteroidal anti-inflammatory agents (Motrin 200-400 mg q6h; Naprosyn 250-375 q6-8h)	Chronic pain is best treated with nonopioid initially (ASA, acetaminophen, ibuprofen, nortriptyline)
	Codeine 30-60 mg q4-6h PO, SC, or IM	Dependence liability for opioids
	Meperidine 50-150 mg q3-4h PO, SC, IM, IV	Side effects of opioids: Sedation, constipation, respiratory depression, nausea, and vomiting
	Methadone 2.5-10 mg q6-8h PO, 10 mg IM	Oral codeine, propoxyphene (Darvon), and pentazocine in usual doses are no more effective than ASA. Morphine, Dilaudid, methadone, levorphanol, fentanyl, and large doses of oxycodone are needed for severe pain
	Dilaudid 2-8 mg q4-8h PO or rectal	
	MS Contin 15-60 mg PO bid	
	Nortriptyline 25-75 mg qd hs	
	Fentanyl patch 25-100 µg/hr	Morphine and other full agonists have no limit on analgesic effectiveness except for limit ascribed to side effects
	Ultram (tramadol) 50-100 mg q4-6h, up to 400 mg/day	
Psychiatric and sleep disorders		
AIDS mania	HAART	Seen in late-stage AIDS
Bipolar (manic depression)	Haloperidol 2.5-10 mg bid Fluphenazine 2-10 mg bid Risperidone 1-4 mg bid Oxanzapine 10-40 mg hs One of above + lithium or divalproex	Must distinguish AIDS mania Care should be directed by a psychiatrist

Anxiety	Buspirone (BuSpar) 5 mg tid	Nonbenzodiazepine-nonbarbiturate; dependence liability negligible; increase dose 5 mg q 2–4 day to effective daily dose of 15–30 mg
Depression	General	Selective serotonin reuptake inhibitors (SSRIs): Advantages are relative safety; well tolerated; fewer drug interactions than tricyclics Disadvantages are sexual dysfunction and increased levels when combined with PIs and NNRTIs Tricyclics: Advantages are utility for also treating neuropathy, insomnia, and diarrhea. Disadvantages are anticholinergic effects and increased tricyclic levels with PIs and NNRTIs
Depression	Fluoxetine (Prozac) 10 mg increasing to average 20 mg qd	Major side effects are nausea, nervousness, insomnia, weight loss, dry mouth, constipation; insomnia may be treated with trazodone Desyrel 25–50 mg hs Increases levels of APV, DLV, EFV, IDV, LPV, NFV, RTV SQV; decreases levels of NVP
	Nortriptyline (Pamelor) 10–25 mg hs increasing to 50–150 mg hs or desipramine (Norpramin) 10–25 mg hs increasing to 50–200 mg hs	Titrate level (>125 ng/dL). Desipramine (>125 ng/dL) both promote sleep and weight gain; increased levels with RTV and LPV
	Sertraline (Zoloft) 25–50 mg qd increasing to 50–150 mg/day	Side effects are similar to those noted for Prozac but are less severe because of shorter half-life; LPV and RTV increase sertraline levels
	Paroxetine (Paxil) 10 mg hs increasing to 20–40 mg/day hs	Promotes sleep; LPV and RTV increase paroxetine level
	Bupropion (Wellbutrin) 100 mg in AM increasing for 150–400 mg/day divided doses	No sexual side effects; and RTV, EFV, and NFV increase bupropion levels, significant is unclear
	Nefazodone (Serzone) 50 mg bid increasing to 300–400 mg/day	Promotes sleep: EFV and IDV levels increased

Table 43. (continued)

Condition	Treatment	Comments
Delirium	Haldol 0.5–1 mg hs Resperidone	
Insomnia	Diphenhydramine (Benadryl) 25–50 mg hs Trazodone (Desyrel) 25–100 mg PO hs Chloral hydrate 500–1000 mg PO hs Ambien 5–10 mg hs	Nonprescription Class IV but often considered one of the safest and least habit-forming sedatives Tolerance with continued use
Apathy	Ritalin 7.5 mg bid with weekly increases until intolerance (hyperactivity), adequate response, or maximum dose (60 mg/day) Pemoline 18.75 mg (1 cap) bid with weekly increases to intolerance (shakiness) or response or maximum dose (150 mg/day or 8 caps)	Utility confirmed for both drugs in HIV-infected patients with fatigue associated with depression and psychological distress (Arch Intern Med 2001;161:411)
Substance abuse	1. Detoxification: Sometimes with long-acting benzodiazepines 2. Treatment of co-morbid conditions: Mental health (depression, bipolar disorder, schizophrenia, personality disorders, etc.), medical conditions, and chronic pain syndromes 3. Maintenance treatment and relapse prevention: Individualized to patient need	
Terminal illness	Morphine or other opioids orally or parenterally; MS Contin PO 15, 30, 60, or 100 mg: usual dose is 15–60 mg PO q12h Patient-controlled analgesia (PCA) for morphine Methadone (previously noted doses) Fentanyl patch	Patients given opioids for acute pain or cancer pain rarely experience euphoria and rarely develop psychic dependence; clinically significant physical dependence develops after several weeks with large doses

9—Drugs Used for HIV-Infected Patients

Table 44. Cost of Drugs Commonly Used in Patients with HIV Infection

Drug	Formulation	Typical Regimen	AWP[a] Unit Price ($)	Cost/Wk ($)	Cost/Yr ($)[b]
Abacavir (Ziagen)	300 mg tab	300 mg PO bid	7.41/300 mg	104	5,400
Acyclovir (Zovirax)	200, 400 mg cap	400 mg PO bid	2.16/400 mg cap	30	1570
	800 mg tab	800 mg PO 4×/day	4.21/800 mg tab	118	—
	500 mg vial	2 g/day IV	35/1 mg vial	515	—
Albendazole (Albenza)	200 mg tab	400–800 mg PO bid	1.49/200 mg tab	42–84	—
Alprazolam (Xanax)	0.25, 0.5, 1, and	0.25–0.5 mg PO bid	0.75/0.50 mg tab	10–20	—
	2 mg tabs				
Amikacin (Amikin)	500 mg vial	500 mg bid IV	47.5/1 g vial	650	—
Amoxicillin	250, 500 mg	500 mg PO tid	0.38/500 mg	8	—
	caps				
Amphotericin B	50 mg vial	50 mg/day IV	20.45/50 mg vial	140	—
Amphotericin lipid complexes					
Abelcet	100 mg vial	5 mg/kg/day IV	240/100 mg	5880	—
AmBisome	100 mg vial	3–5 mg/kg/day IV	392/100 mg	9600	—
Amphotec	100 mg vial	3–4 mg/kg/day IV	186/100 mg	4560	—
Ampicillin	500 mg cap	500 mg PO qid	0.13/500 mg tab	4	—
Amprenavir (Agenerase)	50, 150 mg caps	1200 mg PO bid	1.60/150 mg	180	9318
Atazanavir	200 mg cap	400 mg qd	14.49/200 mg	210	10,920
			cap		
Ativan (Lorazepam)	1 mg tab	1 mg PO bid	0.02/1 mg tab	0.28	—
Atorvastatin	10 mg tab	20 mg/day	2.58/10 mg tab	36	1674
Atovaquone (Mepron)	750 mg/5 mL	750 mg PO bid	775/210 mL	258	—
	250 mg tab	250 mg × 6	7.83/250 mg tab	47	—
Azithromycin (Zithromax)	600 mg tab	1200 mg PO q wk	19.71/600 mg tab	38	—
	500 mg vial	500 mg/day	29.22/500 mg vial	203	7740

193

Table 44. (continued)

Drug	Formulation	Typical Regimen	AWP[a] Unit Price ($)	Cost/Wk ($)	Cost/Yr ($)[b]
AZT	100, 300 mg caps	300 mg bid	6.45/300 mg cap	90	4696
Benadryl (diphenhydramine)	25 mg cap	25 mg HS	0.18/25 mg cap	1	—
Bupropion (Wellbutrin)	150 mg tab	150 mg bid	1.70/150 mg	24	—
Buspar (Buspirone)	5 mg tab	5 mg PO tid	0.91/5 mg tab	19	—
Chloral hydrate	500 mg cap	500 mg hs	0.17/500 mg	1	—
Chlorhexidine (Peridex)	480 mL bottle	Oral rinse bid	10.40/480 mL bottle	—	—
Cidofovir (Vistide)	375 mg/5 mL	5 mg/kg IV q2wk	888/375 mg	444	23,088
Ciprofloxacin (Cipro)	250, 500, 750 mg tabs	500–750 mg PO bid	1.20/500 mg	15	—
Clarithromycin (Biaxin)	400 mg vial	400 mg IV bid	14.41/200 mg vial	403	—
	250, 500 mg tabs	250–500 mg PO bid	4.64/250 mg tab	64	—
			4.64/500 mg tab	64	3328
Clindamycin (Cleocin)	300 mg cap	300 mg PO qid	3.00/300 mg cap	84	—
	300 mg vial	600 mg IV tid	10.41/600 mg vial	218	—
Clotrimazole (Mycelex)	10 mg troche	10 mg PO 5×/day	1.68/10 mg troche	60	3120
Combivir	300 mg AZT + 150 mg 3TC	1 bid	11.42/tab	160	8314
d4T (Stavudine)	15, 20, 30, 40 mg	40 mg bid	6.25/40 mg cap	88	4550
Dapsone	100 mg tab	100 mg PO qd	0.20/100 mg tab	1	65
ddC (HIVID)	0.375 mg tab	0.75 mg PO tid	2.60/0.75 mg tab	55	2883
	0.75 mg tab				
ddI (Videx)	25, 50, 100, 150	400 mg PO hs	4.97/200 mg tab	70	3640
ddI (Videx EC)	125, 200, 250, 400 mg	400 mg/day	11.20/400 mg	77	4004
Delavirdine (Rescriptor)	200 mg tab	400 mg PO tid	1.76/200 mg tab	74	3844
Doxycycline	100 mg cap	100 mg PO bid	1.10/100 mg tab	3	—
Dronabinol (Marinol)	2.5, 5 mg.	2.5–5 mg PO bid	10.52/5 mg	73	3822
Efavirenz (Sustiva)	50, 100, 200 mg caps	600 mg q day	16.17/600 mg cap	113	5886
Emtricitabine (Emtriva)	200 mg caps	200 mg qd	10.10/200 mg	71	3676
Enfuvirude (Fusion)	90 mg vial	90 mg sc bid	34.70/90 mg	486	25260
Erythromycin	250 mg cap	500 mg PO qid	0.18/250 mg cap	4	—
Erythropoietin (Procrit, Epogen)	2000, 3000, 4000, 10,000 unit	10–30,000 units 3×/wk	534/40,000 U	534	—

Drug	Dosage form	Dose	Unit cost		
Ethambutol	400 mg tab	400 mg PO tid	1.78/400 mg tab	38	1?00
	240 mL	240 mL × 4/day	1.50/240 mL	42	1460
Feeding supplements					
Ensure Sustecal, etc.					
Vivonex TEN	1 packet	4 packets/day	6.08/packet	170	8840
Fentanyl patch	µg/hr 25, 50, 75, 100	25 µg/hr q 72 h	12.80/25 µg/hr	26	—
Fenofibrate	48 mg tab	48 mg bid	0.86/48 mg tab	14	728
Fluconazole (Diflucan)	100 mg tab	100 mg PO bid	9.78/100 mg tab[c]	69	—
	400 mg vial	200 mg IV bid	168.83/400mg vial	1176	—
Flucytosine (5 FC)	250, 500mg caps	7600 mg/day	9.02/500 mg	9576	—
Fluoxetine (Prozac)	10, 20 mg caps	10–40 mg/day	2.67/20 mg cap	20–40	—
Flurazepam (Dalmane)	15, 30 mg caps	15–30 mg hs	0.06/30 mg cap	1	—
Fomivirsen	330 µg	330 µg q mo	$880/dose	220	2640
Fosamprenavir (Lexiva)	700 mg tab	1400 mg bid	10.48/700 mg	294	15,288
Saquinavir soft gel caps (Fortovase)	200 mg cap	6 caps tid	1.09/200 mg cap	133	6945
Foscarnet (Foscavir)	6, 12 g vial	6 g IV qd	82.90/6 g vial	581	$30,212
Gammaglobulin (Gamimune, etc)	250 mL vial 5%	60 g IV	800/250 mL vial	2100/dose	—
Ganciclovir (Cytovene)	500 mg vial	350 mg IV qd	38.64/500 mg vial	266	13,832
Gatifloxacin (Tequin)	400 mg	400 mg/day	9.40/400 mg	66	—
G-CSF (Filgrastim, Neupogen)	300, 480 µg vial	75–300 µg IV or SC qd or qod	165.30/300 µg vial	495	—
Gemfibrozil	600 mg vial	600 mg bid	1.24/600 mg tab	16	822
Growth hormone (Serostim)	6 mg vial	6 mg SC/day	252/6 mg vial	1750	—
Triazolam (Halcion)	0.125, 0.25 mg tab	0.25 mg hs	0.78/0.25 mg tab	5	—
Haloperidol (Haldol)	1 mg tab 10, 20 µg/mL	2 mg bid	0.55/1 mg tab	2	160
Hepatitis B vaccine		1 mL SC × 3	156/1 doses	—	—
Hydroxyurea (Hydrea)	500 mg cap	500 mg bid	1.27/500 mg	18	946
Indinavir (Crixivan)	200, 400 mg	800 mg tid	6.21/400 mg cap	175	9027
Interferon-α (Roferon)	3, 6, 9, 18, 36 mil units vial	3–30 mil units IV or SC qd	38.18/36 mil units	220–2200	—
Isoniazid (INH)	300 mg tab	300 mg PO qd	0.16/300 mg tab	1	50
Itraconazole (Sporanox)	100 mg capsule 100 mg/150 mL oral solution	100 mg PO bid 100 mg/day	9.63/100 mg tab 10.71/150 mL	134 1477	6970
Ketoconazole (Nizoral)	200 mg vial 200 mg tab	200 mg day IV 200 mg PO qd	211.91/200 mg 3.09/200 mg tab	1477 25–50	—
Lamivudine (3TC, Epivir)	150 mg tabs	150 mg bid	5.52/150 mg tab	67	3845

Table 44. (continued)

Drug	Formulation	Typical Regimen	AWP[a] Unit Price ($)	Cost/Wk ($)	Cost/Yr ($)[b]
Leucovorin (folinic acid)	5, 10, 15, 25 mg tabs	10 mg PO qd	2.85/5 mg tab	40	2080
Levofloxacin (Levaquin)	250, 500 mg tabs	500 mg PO qd	10.63/500 mg	119	6188
		500 mg IV qd	39.50/500 mg	276	
Lomotil		5 mg PO qid	0.50/2.5 mg tab	18	
Loperamide (Imodium)	2.5 mg tab	2 mg 6 ×/day	0.65/2 mg	27	
Lopinavir/ritonavir (Kaletra)	2 mg cap	3 caps bid	3.76/cap	158	8,234
Lorazepam (Ativan)	133/33 mg caps	1–2 mg tid	1.71/2 mg tab	18	
Megestrol (Megace)	0.5, 1, 2 mg tabs	80 mg PO qid	1.15/40 mg tab	72	
Methadone	20, 40 mg tabs	15–40 mg/day	0.14/10 mg tab	2–3	
Metronidazole	5, 10 mg tabs	250–500 mg PO tid	0.43/250 mg tab	8–16	
	500 mg tab	0.5–1 g IV bid	15.42/500 mg vial	217	
Morphine sulfate (MS Contin)	500 mg vial		1.32/30 mg tab		
Moxifloxacin (Avelox)	30 mg tab	400 mg/day	9.80/400 mg	69	3588
Nelfinavir (Viracept)	250, 625 mg tab	750 mg tid	2.52/250 mg tab	147–160	7644–8320
		1250 mg bid	$6.30/625 mg tab	176	9152
Nevirapine (Viramune)	200 mg tab	200 mg PO bid	6.01/200 mg tab	84	4368
Nortriptyline (Pamelor)	10, 25, 50 mg caps	75 mg PO HS	2.23/75 mg cap	14	
Nystatin	100,000 units/mL	5 u po 5 ×/day	0.11/100,000 units	19	1001
Oxandrolone (Oxandrin)	2.5 mg tab	10–20 mg bid	3.75/2.5 mg	210–420	10,920–21,840
Oxymetholone (Anadrol-50)	50 mg tab	100–350 mg/day	14.88/50 mg tab	207–729	
Paromomycin	250 mg cap	500 mg–1 g bid	3.03/250 mg cap	79–158	
Pegylated interferon	160 µg vial	160 µg/wk	252	252	13,100
Pentamidine	300 mg vial	300 mg aerosolized q mo	98.75/300 mg	25	1200
Pneumovax	0.5 mL vial	0.5 mL × 1 SC or IM	13.42/0.5 mL		11
Pravastatin	10, 20, 40 mg tabs	20–40 mg/day	2.78/20 mg	20–40	1040–2080
Prednisone	50 mg tab	50 mg PO qd	0.22/50 mg tab	2	
Primaquine	15 mg tab	15 mg/day	0.99/15 mg tab	7	
Prozac (fluoxetine)	10, 20 mg pulvule	10–40 mg PO qd	2.67/20 mg	16–32	
Pyrazinamide	500 mg tab	500 mg PO qid	1.12/500 mg tab	31	1612
Pyrimethamine (Daraprim)	25 mg tab	50 mg PO qd	0.55/25 mg tab	7	364

Drug	Preparation	Dose	AWP[a]	Cost/week	Cost/year[b]
Rifabutin (Mycobutin)	150 mg cap	300 mg PO qd	5.77/150 mg cap	80	4150
Rifampin (Rifater)	300 mg cap	600 mg PO qd	1.61/300 mg cap	22	1172
	50 mg INH, 120 mg Rif, 300 mg PZA	1 tab/10 kg/day	1.80/tab	75	—
Ribavirin (Rebetron)	200 mg cap	4–5 caps/day	9.93–11.03/200 mg	280	1560–7800
Methylphenidate (Ritalin)	10 mg tab	10 mg PO tid	0.40/10 mg tab	8	—
Ritonavir (Norvir)	100 mg cap	100–200 mg bid	2.14 or 10.71/100 mg cap[c]	75–150	
Saquinavir	200 mg cap	400 mg PO bid	2.50/200 mg	70	3640
Invirase / Fortovase	200 mg cap	400 mg PO bid	1.33/200 mg	37	2038
Serostim	4, 5, 6 mg vials	6 mg/day SC	42/mg	1764	—
Sulfadiazine	500 mg tab	0.5–2 g qid	1.22/500 mg tab	34–136	5548
Tenofovir (Viread)	300 mg tab	300 mg qd	15.20/300 mg tab	106	500
Testosterone	100 mg/mL 10 mL	200–400 mg IM	1.40/100 mg	10	
Testosterone patch	6 mg/patch	6 mg/day	3.50/patch	24	1238
Trazodone	50, 100, 150, 300 mg tabs	150–300 mg/day	1.41/150 mg tab	30	1500
Triazolam (Halcion)	0.125, 0.25 mg tabs	0.25 mg/d	1.41/0.25 mg tab	5	25
Trimethoprim	100, 200 mg tabs	300 mg tid	0.68/100 mg tab	25	—
Trimethoprim-sulfamethoxazole	DS tab	1–3 DS PO bid	1.21/DS tab	8	416
	SS tab	1 SS PO qd	0.73/SS tab	5	2500
	16/80 mg/mL vial		19.26/30 mL vial	100	
Trizivir	AZT + 3TC + ABC	1 bid	19.40/cap	272	14123
Valganciclovir (Valcyte)	450 mg tab	900 mg/day	31.46/450 mg	440	22880
Vancomycin	125 mg pulvule	125 mg PO qid	6.40/125 mg	155	—
	0.5, 1 g vial	1 g bid IV	5.76/500 mg vial	1528	—
Voriconazole (Vfend)	200 mg tab	200–300 mg PO bid	35/200 mg tab	490	—
	200 mg vial	3–4 mg/kg IV bid	109/200 mg vial	1900	—
Vivonex TEN	1 packet	4 packs PO qd	6.20/packet	173	8996

[a] Average wholesale prices (AWP) from PriceAlert, June 2004.
[b] Annual costs are approximate AWP and restricted to drugs given chronically.
[c] Ritonavir has 2 prices—one is the new AWP at $10.71/100 mg; the second is the prior price of $2.14, which is still used for Medicaid and ADAP. Cost/week and year are given for doses of 200 mg/day

Table 45. Adverse Reactions to Antimicrobial Agents Commonly Used in Patients with HIV Infection

	Frequent	Occasional	Rare
Abacavir (Ziagen)		*Hypersensitivity* reaction with fever, GI symptoms ± cough and rash; usually in 1st 6 wk; this may be a life-threatening complication; frequency is 5% GI intolerance—nausea, malaise, diarrhea, anorexia	Lactic acidosis and hepatic steatofosis (class adverse reaction that is rare with ABC)*
Acyclovir (Zovirax)	Initiation at infusion site (IV infusion)	Nausea and vomiting; diarrhea Nephrotoxicity with high doses IV, prior renal disease, and other nephrotoxic durgs	CNS toxicity (dose-related, usually with rapid IV infusion, prior renal failure, or concurrent nephrotoxic drugs) agitation, encephalopathy, disorientation, seizures; hallucinations; Marrow: anemia: neutropenia; thrombocytopenia; Miscellaneous: hypotension; rash; renal toxicity especially with prior renal disease; hepatotoxicity; pruritis
Albendazole (Eskazole)		Hepatotoxicity, reversible neutropenia—monitor CBC and liver function tests	GI intolerance: hypersensitivity; neutropenia; dizziness; hair loss (reversible)
Aminoglycosides Tobramycin Gentamicin Amikacin Netilmicin Kanamycin	Renal failure—dose related; monitor creatinine ≥3×/wk Once daily dosing does not increase toxicity	Vestibular and auditory toxicity—dose related Monitor Romberg and reading after rapid head motion; warn patient to report ear fullness and decreased hearing or dizziness	Fever; rash; blurred vision; neuromuscular blockage; eosinophilia

Amphotericin
Amphotericin B/lipid formulations (CID 2002;44:63)

Formulations	Frequent — Creatinine ↑ 2× over baseline (1%)	Occasional — chills (%)	Rare — Infusion-related fewer > 1°C (%)
Amphotericin B	30–50	55	40
Abelcet	15–20	15–20	10–20
Amphotec	10–25	30–50	10–20
AmBisome	20	20	7

Drug	Frequent	Occasional	Rare
Amprenavir (Agenerase)	GI intolerance nausea—5% diarrhea—15% Rash—11% Oral paresthesias—28% Class adverse reactions*	Hepatotoxicity	Liquid preparation is 55% propylene glycol—seizures, stupor, lactic acidosis, renal failure, hemolysis (This form is contraindicated in pregnancy; renal failure, or hepatic failure)
Atazanavir (Reyataz)	Drug malabsorption with reduced acid Increased indirect bilirubinemia—is inocuous but causes clinical jaundice in 7% Class reactions except hyperlipidemia	GI intolerance Increased transaminase levels	Increased QTc and/or PR interval
Atorvastatin (Lipitor)		Myopathy with muscle pain, CPK increase ± fever Hepatitis 1–2% Miscellaneous—diarrhea, nausea, dizziness headache, insomnia	Rhabdomyolysis + renal failure Impotence
Atovaquone (Mepron)	Rash (20%), nausea (20%), diarrhea (20%); these are sufficiently severe to require discontinuation in 9%	Vomiting, pruritis	Headache, fever, insomnia

Table 45. (continued)

	Frequent	Occasional	Rare
Azithromycin (Zithromax)		GI intolerance (dose related) (6%); Diarrhea (4%), reversible ototoxicity (2%), skin rash (1%), headache, fatigue, drowsiness (1%)	Erythema multiforme; increased transaminase Pseudomembranous colitis
Benzodiazepines	Dependency, tolerance, and withdrawal reactions (related to dose and duration); Daytime sedation, dizziness, ataxia, incoordination Amnesia for events during drug's time of action	Blurred vision, diplopia, confusion, memory disturbance, fatigue, incontinence, constipation, hypotension, bizarre behavior	
Bupropion (Wellbutrin)	Weight loss	Agitation, insomnia GI intolerance with anorexia, nausea, vomiting	Psychosis, paranoia depersonalization
Buspirone (BuSpar)	CNS: Dizziness, headache, sedation (10%); warn patient	Psychomotor dysfunction, fatigue, anxiety, insomnia (5%); nausea (6-8%); depression (3%); dream disturbance; GI—dry mouth, constipation, diarrhea (1-5%); tachycardia (2%); sexual dysfunction	
Cephalosporins	Phlebitis at infusion sites; diarrhea (especially cefoperazone); pain at IM injection sites (less with cefazolin)	Allergic reactions (anaphylaxis rare); Diarrhea and colitis including C. difficile-associated colitis and PMC; eosinophilia, positive Coombs' test	Hemolytic anemia; Interstitial nephritis (cephalothin), hepatic dysfunction, convulsions (high dose with renal failure), neutropenia, hypoprothrombinemia (cefamandole, cefoperazone, and cefotetan)

Cidofovir (Vistide)	*Renal failure*—25% develop ≥2 + proteinuria or creatinine increase >2–3 mg/dL (reversible if discontinued). Monitor creatinine and urine protein at baseline and 48 hr prior to each dose Must pretreat with IV hydration and probenecid. Probenecid side effects in AIDS patients in 50%: Fever, rash, headache, nausea, GI Rx intolerance—reduce with antiemetics, antipyretics, or antihistamines (Ann Intern Med 1997;126:257) Neutropenia in 15%; monitor CBC	Fanconi syndrome: proteinuria, hypophosphatemia, hypouracemia, glycosuria, and decreased serum bicarbonate GI intolerance: Give antiemetics	Ocular hypotony, anterior uveitis, iritis
Ciprofloxacin (see quinolones)			
Clarithromycin (Biaxin)		GI intolerance (3%), headache (2%), antibiotic-associated diarrhea	Pseudomembraneous colitis
Clindamycin (Cleocin)	Diarrhea (10–30%)	Nausea, vomiting, anorexia morbilliform, rash, pruritis, C. difficile-associated colitis or PMC	Stevens-Johnson syndrome: Joint pains, neutropenia, thrombocytopenia
Clotrimazole (Lotrimin, Mycelex, etc.)		Oral—increased transaminase (15%), nausea and vomiting (5%). Topical (skin and vaginal)—rash, burning, pruritus	

Table 45. (continued)

	Frequent	Occasional	Rare
Dapsone	Rash, fever, nausea, anorexia, neutropenia—sufficiently severe to require discontinuation in up to 30–40%	Hemolytic anemia—Methemoglobinemia with dyspnea, cyanosis, fatigue, tachycardia and chocolate-colored blood. This is dose and duratin—related and may or may not be related to G-6-PD deficiency. Laboratory tests—increased indirect bilirubin and LDH with smear showing spherocytes. Methemoglobulin levels <25% are usually tolerated except with concurrent lung disease. If severe—treat with O_2 and RBCs ± activated charcoal ± methylene blue (if no G-6-PD deficiency) (JAIDS 1996;12:477).	Hypoalbuminemia; epidermal necrolysis; optic atrophy; aplastic anemia; agranulocytosis; peripheral neuropathy; aplastic anemia; "suffone syndrome"—fever, exfoliative dermatitis, jaundice, adenopathy, methemoglobinemia, and anemia—treat with steroids; nephrosis; allergic reactions, insomnia, irritability, headache (transient), blurred vision, ringing in ears, hepatitis
Daunorubicin (DaunoXome)	Granulocytopenia—monitor CBC predose. Triad of flushing, back pain, and chest tightness—14%; follows infusions and resolves with discontinuation or slowing of infusion	Cardiotoxicity especially with prior cardiac disease or prior treatment with anthracyclines. Monitor ejection fraction with use of large doses ($\geq$320 mg/m^2)	Extravasation—tissue necrosis
Delavirdine (Rescriptor)	Rash (18%) maculopapular red, upper body; 4% require drug discontinuation	Headaches Hepatitis	Erythema multiforme, Stevens-Johnson syndrome

Drug		
Didanosine (ddI; Videx)	GI intolerance 15–20%—diarrhea nausea, vomiting bloating—significantly reduced with Videx EC; *Pancreatitis* (1–9%)—risk is increased with concurrent d4T or history of EtOH, prior pancreatitis, low CD4 count *Peripheral neuropathy* (5–12%)—rate increased with high total dose, use with d4T. Note: Na^{++} load of 265 mg/tab and 1350 mg/powder packet	Class ADRs—Lactic acidosis, steatosis, lipoatrophy* (Avoid concurrent d4T/ddI when possible)	Rash, hyperuricemia, hypokalemia; hypomagnesemia: optic neuritis; marrow suppression
Dideoxycytidine (ddC; HIVID)	Peripheral neuropathy 17–31%, frequency is related to cumulative dose Avoid concurrent d4T or ddI	Aphthous ulcers, rash, pancreatitis (<1%); hepatitis Flulike complaints Class ADR—Lactic acidosis, steatosis, lipoatrophy*	Thrombocytopenia, leukopenia
Doxycycline	GI intolerance (10%), nausea ± diarrhea (reduced with food), dysphagia Photosensitivity, *Candida* vaginitis Deposited in developing teeth—avoid in midpregnancy to term and children <8 yr		Rash
Dronabinol (Marinol)	Dose-related mood high; somnolence, confusion (usually resolves with continued use in 1–3 day) GI intolerance in 3–10% Dizziness in 3–10%	Abuse potential, especially with substance abusers, elderly patients with psychiatric illness, and those receiving sedatives, hypnotics, etc.	Hypotension, vasodilation asthenia, tachycardia, visual disturbances, asthenia

Table 45. (continued)

	Frequent	Occasional	Rare
Efavirenz (Sustiva)	CNS toxicity (53%) with abnormal dreams, confusion, depersonalization, dizziness; usually resolves in 3 wk. Rash (15–27%)—morbilliform, usually in first 14 day; requires discontinuation in 2% Lipids—increased triglyceride and cholesterol including HDL, cholesterol (JID 2004; 189:1056)	Hepatotoxicity with elevated transaminase levels in 2–8% False positive test for cannabinoid (marijuana)	Stevens-Johnson syndrome
EPO (epogen, Procrit)		Headache, arthralgias, flulike illness, GI intolerance, diarrhea, fatigue, edema	Hypertension, seizures (?)
Erythromycin	GI intolerance (oral-dose related): Phlebitis (IV)	Diarrhea, stomatitis, cholestatic hepatitis (especially estolate reversible) Generalized rash	Allergic reactions, colitis, hemolytic anemia, reversible ototoxicity (especially with high doses and renal failure) Ventricular arrhythmics
Emtricitabine (Emtriva)		GI intolerance—1% require discontinuation Skin hyperpigmentation	Class adverse reactions: lactic acidosis—rare with FTC*
Enfuvirtide (Fuseon)	Injection site reaction with pain (9%), pruritis (62%), induration (89%), erythema (32%), and nodules (26%)—Reduce by rotating injection sites	Bacterial pneumonia rates are increased 5× for unexplained reasons	GI intolerance; hypotension; elevated transaminase; glomerulonephritis; chills and fever; marrow suppression; Guillain-Barre syndrome; Bell's palsy; pancreatitis hyperglycemia (Relationship to drug is unclear for most of these ADRs

Drug		
Ethambutol (Myambutol)	Optic neuritis: Decreased acuity, reduced color discrimination, constricted fields, scotomata—dose related and infrequent with ≤20 mg/kg/day Patients given ≥25 mg/kg/d should have baseline visual acuity and red-green color perception test; repeat monthly	Hypersensitivity: Peripheral neuropathy, GI intolerance, thrombocytopenia, toxic epidermal neurolysis, lichenoid skin rash
Fenofibrate (Tricor)	Hepatotoxicity in 6%, dose related Flulike syndrome Rash, pruritis ± urticaria in 1–3% Myositis with muscle pain and increased CPK	Pancreatitis; cholecystitis; agranulocytosis; thrombocytopenia: eczema
Fentanyl patch	Central nervous system depression and respiratory depression—especially in opiate-naive patients: dose related Tolerance with extended courses Local side effects: Erythema, pruritis, edema at site of application	
Fluconazole (Diflucan)	Reversible alopecia in 10–20% receiving ≥400 mg/day for >3 mo (Ann Intern Med 1995;123:354)	GI tolerance 1.5–8% Rash 5% Hepatitis with inreased ALT to >8 × ULN in 1% Miscellaneous—dizziness, hypokalemia and headache in 2%

Additional column (rightmost):

Fluconazole (Diflucan)	Stevens-Johnson syndrome, thrombocytopenia, anaphylaxis, hypokalemia

Table 45. (continued)

	Frequent	Occasional	Rare
Flucytosine (Ancobon)	GI intolerance (including nausea, vomiting, diarrhea, and ulcer-active colitis)	Marrow suppression with leukopenia or thrombocytopenia (dose related, especially with renal failure, level > 100 μg/mL or concurrent amphotericin): Monitor WBC, avoid dose > 100 mg/kg/d, and maintain peak serum level at 50–100 μg/mL. Miscellaneous: confusion; rash; hepatitis (dose related)	Hallucinations, eosinophilia, granulocytosis, fatal hepatitis, peripheral neuropathy
Fluoxetine (Prozac)	GI intolerance (20%), anorexia, weight loss, nausea CNS (20%)—anxiety, agitation, insomnia, sexual dysfunction	Headache, tremor, drowsiness, dry mouth, sweating, diarrhea, skin rash	Acute dystonia, akathisia (sensation of motor restlessness); possible suicidal ideation (included as package insert warning required by FDA)
Fosamprenavir (Lexiva)	Skin rash in 12–33%; must discontinue drug in <1% GI intolerance in up to 40%; severe in 5–10%	Elevated transaminase levels in 6–8% Class adverse reactions*	
Foscarnet (Foscar)	Dose-related renal failure or renal failure (reversible)—30% get creatinine >2 mg/dL Monitor creatinine 1–3×/wk and discontinue if creatinine clearance <0.4 mL/min/kg or creatinine >2.9 mg/dL	Electrolyte changes—reduced Ca^{++}, ionized Ca^{++} Mg^{++}, PO_4^-, K^+ (8–16%) (monitor electrolytes 1–2×/wk and symptoms—paresthesias and numbness); ionized calcium; Seizures—10% related to renal failure and hypocalcemia Miscellaneous—penile ulcers; nausea relieved with slowing infusion or antinausea agent	Headache; rash; fever; marrow suppression; hepatitis

Drug		
G-CSF (Neupogen, Filgrastim)	Bone pain in 10–20% (usually controlled with acetaminophen)	Erythema or pain at injection site	Anemia, thrombocytopenia, wheezing, acute febrile dermatosis (Sweet's syndrome), vasculitis
Ganciclovir (Cytovene)	*Neutropenia* with absolute neutrophil count <1000/mm³ in 25–50%. Monitor CBC 2–3×/wk and discontinue if ANC <500/mm³ or platelet count <25,000/mm³; dose related	Thrombocytopenia (2–8%); anemia (2%); fever; rash; CNS toxicity with headaches, seizure confusion in 10–15% Miscellaneous—abnormal liver function tests (2%); renal failure	Psychosis; neuropathy; impaired reproductive function (?); nausea; vomiting; GI bleeding or perforation; myocardiopathy; encephalopathy
Gemfibrozil		Gallstones secondary to cholesterol excretion GI intolerance Increase LDL cholesterol	Marrow suppression
Growth hormone (Serostim)	Musculoskeletal discomfort 20–50% Swelling hands and feet in up to 25%—resolves with continued treatment Fat atrophy	Increased insulin resistance—diabetes Miscellaneous—flulike symptoms, rigors, back pain, carpal tunnel syndrome, chest pain, nausea, diarrhea (most are dose related)	
Haloperidol (Haldol)	CNS: Extrapyramidal symptoms	CNS: Dystonia, motor restlessness; tardive dyskinesia (abrupt withdrawal); sexual dysfunction (10–20%)	Neuroleptic malignant syndrome; hypotension; hepatitis

Table 45. (continued)

	Frequent	Occasional	Rare
Hydroxyurea (Hydrea)	Leukopenia and/or anemia—reverses when treatment is discontinued; Increases risk of pancreatitis and peripheral neuropathy when used with ddI ± d4T (Must use with ddI)	GI intolerance: Rashes—maculopapular rash, facial erythema, hyperpigmentation, oral ulceration; Chronic leg ulcers with use >3 yr;	Dysuria, hyperuricemia, renal failure, disorientation; hallucinations; drowsiness; seizures; chills, fever, alopecia, pancreatitis
Ibuprofen	GI intolerance (give with milk); increased transaminase levels—15%	Peptic ulcer: Bleed or perforation; CNS—dizziness, headache, anxiety; tinnitis	Aseptic meningitis, amblyopia, hearing loss; severe liver toxicity; marrow suppression; renal failure; anaphylaxis
Indinavir (Crixivan)	Asymptomatic increase in indirect bilirubinemia (10–15%) ascribed to precipitation of drug in renal system—related to state of hydration and peak IDV levels. Monitor for symptoms, obtain urinalysis and creatinine of 3 mo and reduce risk with ≥48 oz fluids/day (JAIDS 2003;32: 135)	Interstitial nephritis—2% (CID 2002;34:1033) GI intolerance Transaminase elevation Skin, hair and nails: Reversible alopecia, sicca syndrome with dry skin and mucous membranes; paronychia Class ADRs with insulin resistance, increased lipids, fat accumulation*	Metallic taste, fatigue, insomnia, blurred vision, dizziness, rash, thrombocytopenia, fulminant hepatic failure
Interferon-α (Roferon, Intron)	Flu-like (80% with 35 mil units/d)—fever, fatigue, anorexia, headache, myalgics; depression—reduce with NSAIDs; GI intolerance (20–65%)—nausea, vomiting, abdominal pain, diarrhea Hepatotoxicity: 10–50% Rash 25%	CNS toxicity; Confusion, paresthesias, concentration problems; amnesia; Miscellaneous—pruritis; marrow supression; alopecia; proteinuria	Delirium, obtundation

Drug			
Isoniazid (INH)	Hepatitis—rate increases with age and abuse of alcohol; incidence of increase to >5× general population and 2.6% with ETOH or elderly (Ann Intern Med 1999;181:1014); warn patient; clinical evaluation monthly; D/C if ALT/AST ≥5× ULN; get baseline LFT and repeat prn	Allergic reactions; fever; peripheral Peripheral neuropathy—reduce with pyridoxine 50 mg/day; risk increased with diabetes, ETOH, pregnancy malnutrition, or AIDS Miscellaneous—rash, fever, adenopathy, GI intolerance	CNS—optic neuritis, psychosis, convulsions, myocardiopathy, encephalopathy, blood dyscrasia, lupus like syndrome, keratitis, pellagra-like rash
Itraconazole (Sporanox)	Negative inotropic effect (new FDA black box warning); GI intolerance (5–10%); Rash (1–9%)	Hepatitis in 4%: monitor LFTs Miscellaneous—pruritus, hypertension, hypokalemia, edema	Fulminant hepatitis (1:1000 and reversible) Ventricular fibrillation
Ketoconazole (Nizoral)	GI intolerance (dose related);	Temporary increase in transaminase levels (2–5%), Endocrine—decreased steroid and testosterone synthesis with impotence, gynecomastia, oligospermia, reduced libido; menstrual abnormalities (prolonged use and dose related, usually ≥600 mg/day) Miscellaneous—headache; dizziness; asthenia; pruritus; rash	Abrupt hepatitis (1:15,000): rare cases of fatal hepatic necrosis; anaphylaxis; lethargy; arthralgias; fever; marrow suppression; hypothyroidism (genetically determined); thrombocytopenia; hallucinations
Lamivudine (3TC, Epivir)		Headache, nausea, diarrhea, abdominal pain, insomnia	Pancreatitis—reported in pediatric pts, ? in adults Class ADRs—lactic acidosis ± steatosis that is rare with 3TC*

Table 45. (continued)

	Frequent	Occasional	Rare
Levofloxacin (Levaquin)—see quinolones			
Megestrol acetate (Megace)		Sexual dysfunction (estrogen—may respond to testosterone); Hyperglycemia—5% Adrenal insufficiency or Cushing's syndrome (Arch Intern Med 1997;157:1651) Miscellaneous—diarrhea; rash; asthenia; flatulence; pain; GI intolerance;	Carpal tunnel syndrome, thrombosis, vaginal bleeding, alopecia, high dose (480–1600 mg/day)—chest pressure, hypertension, dyspnea, congestive heart failure
Lopinavir/ritonavir (Kaletra)	GI intolerance with diarrhea in 15–25% usually controlled with Imodium	Transaminase level increase with ALT to 5× ULN in 10–12% Class ADRs with insulin resistance, increased lipids and visceral fat increase*	Renal and parotid lithiasis (AIDS 2004;18:705)
Metronidazole (Flagyl)	GI intolerance, metallic taste	Peripheral neuropathy (prolonged use—usually reversible); Phlebitis at injection sites; Antabuse-like reaction with alcohol ingestion Miscellaneous—headache furry tongue	Seizures; ataxic encephalitis; leukopenia; dysuric; pancreatitis; allergic reactions; mutagenic in Ames test (clinical relevance as carcinogen with long-term use is unclear); hypotension; ataxia; coma; somnolence; C. difficile-associated colitis

Morphine + other opiate agonists	Tolerance, physical dependence, psychological dependence, withdrawal syndrome (slight with 80 mg MS/d × 30 day; severe with 240 mg MS/day × 30 day)	Acute toxicity: Coma, respiratory depression, cardiac arrest
Nelfinavir (Viracept)	Diarrhea—10–30%; usually controlled with imodium or calcium (Tums)—sufficiently severe to require discontinuation in 1.6%	Class adverse reactions: Insulin resistance, increased lipids and visceral fat accumulation*
Nevirapine (Viramune)	Rash (17–30%) usually maculopapular and erythematous ± pruritis usually in first 8 wk; discontinue if rash is severe, accompanied by fever, blisters, or mucous membrane involvement Hepatotoxicity with hepatic necrosis and possibly death even if NDV is stopped; most common in first 8–16 wk in treatment-naïve women with CD4 count >250 (11%); often presents with drug rash, eosinophilia, and systemic symptoms (DRESS Syndrome) Avoid NVP as initial treatment in women with CD4 count >250 and men with CD4 count >400; monitor LFTs in first 3 mo.	Nausea	Fever, headache Stevens-Johnson syndrome, three rash reactions associated with death (Lancet 1998;351:567)

Table 45. (continued)

	Frequent	Occasional	Rare
	Second form of hepatotoxicity (in 10–15%); transamination elevations, which occurs later in treatment, is usually asymptomatic, appears similar to transaminase elevation seen with PIs and EFV; this is often reversible even if NVP is continued; some D/C NVP if ALT is >5–10 × ULN		
Nortriptyline and other tricyclics (Pamelor, Aventyl)	Anticholinergic activity; dry mucous membranes, blurred vision, constipation, urinary retention; CNS: Drowsiness, weakness, fatigue, sexual dysfunction	Extrapyramidal symptoms: Tremor, rigidity, dystonia, dysarthria. Miscellaneous—increased transaminase levels; weight gain; sexual dysfunction; orthostatic hypotension	Neuroleptic malignant syndrome, peripheral neuropathy, ataxia marrow suppression, hepatitis arrhythmias
Nystatin (Mycostatin)		GI intolerance (nausea, vomiting, diarrhea)	
Oxandrolone (Oxandrin)	Virilization in women	Hepatic toxicity with cholestatic hepatitis; monitor LFTs. Miscellaneous—GI intolerance, ankle swelling, insomnia, depression	Peliosis hepatitis (blood-filled hepatic cysts)

Drug			
Oxymetholone (Anadrol-50)	Cholestatic jaundice Miscellaneous—GI intolerance Decreased TSH and T4		Hepatic necrosis Peliosis hepatis Hepatic cancer Intra-abdominal hemorrhage Osteoporosis
Paromomycin (Humatin)	GI intolerance, steatorrhea, and malabsorption		Rash, headache, vertigo Aminoglycoside: With GI absorption ± renal failure there could be nephrotoxicity or ototoxicity
Pegylated interferon (PegIntron, Pegasys)	CNS—depression in 21–29%—caution with history of psychiatric disorder Marrow suppression PMN <500 in 1% Platelets <20,000 in 1% Flulike symptoms—38%; Rx NSAIDS, ASA, etc. Injection site reaction—47% pain, pruritis, etc. GI intolerance: 15–30% Alopecia: 20%; pruritis: 10%; rash: 6%	Thyroiditis with hyper- or hypothyroidism; monitor TSH q 12 wk Retinopathy especially with diabetes, HBP, etc. Pruritis and rash 6–10%	Suicide, cardiac arrhythmias; colitis; pancreatitis; hypersensitivity disorders; hepatitis; diabetes

Table 45. (continued)

	Frequent	Occasional	Rare
Penicillins		Hypersensitivity reactions: Rash (especially ampicillin and amoxicillin). Diarrhea (especially ampicillin, amoxicillin) C. difficile—associated diarrhea especially with expanded spectrum agents (amoxicillin, piperacillin etc.) GI intolerance (oral agents); Miscellaneous—fever, Coombs' test positive; phlebitis at infusion sites and sterile abscesses at IM sites; Jarisch-Herxheimer reaction (syphilis or other spirochetal infections)	Anaphylaxis; leukopenia thrombocytopenia; colitis (especially ampicillin) hepatic damage; renal damage; seizures; twitching (high doses in patients with renal failure); hyperkalemia (penicillin G infusion); abnormal platelet aggregation with bleeding diathesis (carbenicillin and ticarcillin)
Pentamidine (Pentam)	Nephrotoxicity (25%); usually 2nd week of treatment and usually reversible (CID 1997; 24;854) Monitor renal function	Hypotension in 6% (especially with rapid infusions; infuse ≥60 min and monitor BP) Hypoglycemia (5–10%), usually after 1 wk, may last days with glucose <25 mg/dL; hyperglycemia in 2–9% and insulin-dependent diabetes; GI intolerance: Nausea, vomiting, abdominal pain, anorexia, and/or bad taste; Marrow suppression with leukopenia or thrombocytopenia 2–13%	Hepatotoxicity, leukopenia, thrombocytopenia, pancreatitis, hypocalcemia, rash, pruritis, fever, urticaria, anaphylaxis, toxic epidermal necrolysis

Drug			
	Aerosol administration—cough (in 30%—prevent with Albuterol 2 puffs). Note: risk of TB transmission	Aerosol administration—asthma reaction (in 5%—prevent with Albuterol, 2 puffs), laryngitis, chest pain	
Phenytoin (Dilantin)	Blood levels >25 μg/mL—nystagmus, ataxia, diplopia; >30 μg/mL—lethargy; >50—extreme lethargy	GI intolerance: Gingival hypertrophy; rash; fever; lymphadenopathy. Blood levels >25 μg/mL: Hypotension, sexual dysfunction; hepatitis. Laboratory tests: Prothrombin time increased, positive LE prep, glucose increased, calcium decreased, thyroid hormones T3 and T4 increased	Dyskinesias, marrow suppression, periarteritis nodosa, acute psychosis
Pravastatin (Pravachol)		Myopathy with muscle pain and increased CPK. Hepatitis with ALT increase in 1–2%. Miscellaneous—GI intolerance, rash	Rhabdomyolysis, Impotence
Primaquine		Hemolytic anemia (G-6-PD deficiency)—warn patient to observe for dark urine and/or screen with G-6-PD level pretreatment; GI intolerance—give with meals	Headache, pruritus, Methemoglobinemia, hypertension, arrhythmias, disturbed visual accommodation

Table 45. (continued)

	Frequent	Occasional	Rare
Pyrazinamide (PZA)	Nongouty polyarthralgia. 40% Asymptomatic hyperuricemia use with caution with history of gout	Hepatitis (dose related). Short course (2 mo) PZA + rifabutin regimen for latent TB was associated with high rate of hepatitis including deaths due to fulminant hepatic failure. Monitor LFTs (Am J Respir Crit Care Med 2003;167:1472)	Rash, fever, porphyria, photosensitivity, acute yellow atrophy of liver, acne, skin discoloration, pruritis, sideroblastic anemia, thrombocytopenia
Pyrimethamine (Daraprim)		Folic acid deficiency with megaloblastic anemia and pancytopenia (dose related and reversed with leucovorin) Allergic reactions (primarily with Fansidar) GI intolerance (reduce dose or give with meals)	CNS—ataxia, tremors, seizures, (dose related), fatigue, headache, depression, insomnia
Quinolones	Animal studies show arthropathies in weightbearing joints of immature animals; significance in humans is unknown, but this class is considered contraindicated in children and during pregnancy	GI intolerance (1–5%); CNS—headache, malaise, insomnia, dizziness Allergic reactions; rash (mild and transient in 1–4%) Candida vaginitis; Miscellaneous—tendon rupture, prolonged QT interval (rare but important)	Papilledema; nystagmus; visual disturbances; PMC; abnormal LFTs including hepatic necrosis; marrow suppression; photosensitivity; anaphylaxis; seizures; toxic psychosis; CNS stimulation—tremors, restlessness, confusion; arthralgias; interstitial nephritis; renal failure

Ribavirin (Rebetron)	Anemia—hemolytic in first wk, stabilizes by wk 4; monitor CBC—may need to D/C or give EPO	Nucleoside—may promote side effects of NRTIs, especially ddl Miscellaneous—leukopenia, increased bilirubin, increased uric acid; dyspnea
Rifabutin (Mycobutin)	Red-brown discoloration of secretions (tears, sweat, stool, saliva, skin)	Uveitis—dose related presentation—blurring, photophobia, floaters (NEJM 1994;330:438) Rash—4% GI intolerance—3% Neutropenia—2%	Flulike illness, hepatitis, hemolysis, thrombocytopenia, myositis
Rifampin	Red-brown discoloration of urine, tears (contact lenses), sweat	Hepatitis (cholestatic-changes usually in 1st mo of treatment—frequency not inreased when given with INH); jaundice (usually reversible); GI intolerance; Hypersensitivity reactions (especially with intermittent use); CNS: headache, fatigue, confusion, especially in 1st weeks of treatment; Induces cytochrome P-450 to reduce drug levels (see drug interactions); Flulike symptoms in 0.4–0.7% given RIF 2×/wk characterized by fever, aches ± dyspnea, wheezing	Thrombocytopenia, leukopenia, eosinophilia, hemolytic anemia, renal damage, proximal myopathy, hyperuricemia, anaphylaxis

Table 45. (continued)

	Frequent	Occasional	Rare
Ritonavir (Norvir)	GI intolerance—(nausea, anorexia, abdominal pain noted in most given standard dose) Hyperlipidemia with increased cholesterol and triglycerides (dose related) Extensive drug interactions	Circumoral and peripheral paresthesias. Hepatitis: more common cause of transaminase increases compared to other PIs—dose-related (JAMA 2000;238:74; CID 2000;31: 1234) Class ADRs: Insulin resistance, hyperlipidemia, and visceral fat increase*	Hyperuricemia
Saquinavir (Fortovase)	GI intolerance (nausea, diarrhea, abdominal pain—20–30% of recipients of Fortovase and 5–15% of recipients of Invirase), dose related, less with Invirase	Class adverse reactions: Insulin resistance, hyperlipidemia, and visceral fat accumulation Hepatitis	Headache, thrombocytopenia, rash
Stavudine (d4T; Zerit)	Peripheral neuropathy (15–21%), dose related; increased with concurrent ddl Lactic acidosis ± hepatic steatosis Fat atrophy Macrocytosis (inconsequential)	Pancreatitis (0.5–1%), increased pancreatitis when given with ddl GI intolerance, headache	Hepatotoxicity, esophageal ulcers

Drug		
Sulfonamides	Rash, pruritus, fever, leukopenia	Erythema multiforme, Stevens-Johnson syndrome Myocarditis; psychosis; neuropathy; dizziness; depression; hemolytic anemia (G-6-PD deficiency); marrow suppression; ogranulocytosis; photosensitivity
Tenofovir (Viread)	Crystalluria with renal damage, urolithiasis, and oliguria—dose related and prevented with high output or alkaline urine; GI intolerance; Hemolytic anemia with G-6PD deficiency	GI intolerance, especially flatulance Fanconi syndrome—primarily in patients given standard dose with renal insufficiency. Note: hypophosphatemia, hypouricemia, proteinuria, englycemic glycosuria (JAIDS 2004;35:269; AIDS 2004;18: 960)
Testosterone (IM)	Androgenic (and anabolic) effects—acne, flushing, virilizing to women, gynecomastia, increased libido, priapsim, edema	Cholestatic hepatitis Aggravation of sleep apnea, salt retention
Thalidomide (Thalomid)	100% teratogenic when given at days 35–50 of pregnancy (J Am Acad Dermatol 1996; 35:969) Drowsiness (insomnia was the former indication) Fever and rash in 36%	Dose related paresthesias and extremity pain (may be irreversible); Neutropenia Constipation Dizziness, mood changes, bradycardia, bitter taste, pruritus, hypotension Stevens-Johnson syndrome

Table 45. (continued)

	Frequent	Occasional	Rare
Trazodone (Desyrel)	Sedation in 15–20%	Orthostatic hypotension (5%) Anticholinergic effects—less compared with tricyctics Nervousness, fatigue, dizziness, agitation	Priapism (1/6000)
Trimethoprim	Hyperkalemia in 20–50% given >15 mg/kg/day (NEJM 1993; 328:703). GI intolerance (dose related)	Marrow: Megaloblastic anemia, neutropenia, thrombocytopenia, Rash (3%)	Pancytopenia
Trimethoprim-sulfamethoxazole (Bactrim, Septra)	*Fever, pruritis, rash* (AIDS patients: 30–40% required discontinuation, but 60–70% tolerate drug with readministration; dose related)	GI intolerance: Nausea, vomiting, anorexia, diarrhea including C. difficile-associated colitis Candida vaginitis; Hepatitis including cholestatic jaundice; Marrow—anemia ± G6PD deficiency, thrombocytopenia; neutropenia;	Renal failure, erythema multiforme; anemia; thrombocytopenia Ataxis, apathy, ankle clonus, Stevens-Johnson syndrome, erythema multiforme; urticaria, exfoliative dermittis; Pancreatitis; hepatic necrosis

Drug			
Vancomycin	Phlebitis at injection site	"Red-man syndrome": Flushing ± dyspnea, urticaria, pruritis, and/or wheezing ascribed to histamine release and directly related to rate of infusion—treat with slowing infusion ± antihistamines, corticosteroids, and/or IV fluids Eosinophilia; allergic reactions with rash; Phlebites at infusion sites	Anaphylaxis; ototoxicity and ? nephrotoxicity (dose related); peripheral neuropathy; marrow suppression
Voriconazole (Vfend)	Visual effects in 30%; reversible; decreased vision, color changes, photophobia—warn patient & treat through	Rash—6% Hepatitis—increased ALT in 13%, usually resolves with continued treatment, monitor ALT	Stevens-Johnson syndrome, erythema multiforme
Zidovudine (AZT, Retrovir)	Marrow suppression with anemia or leukopenia related to dose, reversible with discontinuation and/or G-CSF or EPO. Monitor CBC and discontinue with Hgb <8 g/dL or ANC <750/mm³. Macrocytosis (inconsequential) Nail pigmentation (inconsequential)	Subjective complaints with headache, flu-like symptoms, insomnia, asthenia, and/or myalgias—dose related; GI intolerance—especially nausea, altered taste Class ADRs—lactic acidosis* Myopathy and cardiomyopathy—role of AZT is often unclear	Seizures (reversible): Allergy (rash, anaphylaxis); twitching; mania; hepatitis; cardiomyopathy (ECHO shows decrease EF)

* Class adverse reactions with antiretroviral agents: See pg 102–107

Table 46. Drug Interactions

Drug	Effect of Interaction
Abacavir: None	
Acyclovir	
Narcotics	Increased meperidine levels
Probenecid	Increased acyclovir levels
Albendazole: None	
Amphotericin B	
Aminoglycosides	Increased nephrotoxicity[a]
Capreomycin	Increased nephrotoxicity[a]
Cisplatin	Increased nephrotoxicity
Corticosteroids	Increased hypokalemia
Cyclosporine	Increased nephrotoxicity
Digitalis	Increased cardiotoxicity (monitor K^+)
Diuretics	Increased hypokalemia
Methoxyflurane	Increased nephrotoxicity
Skeletal muscle relaxants	Increased effect of relaxants
Vancomycin	Increased nephrotoxicity
Amprenavir and Fosamprenavir (Inhibits cytochrome P-450 CYP 3A4 enzymes)	
Abacavir	Increases ABC levels 30%—standard doses
Astemizole	Ventricular arrhythmias[a]
Bepridil	Increased bepridil levels[a]
Warfarin (Coumadin)	Increased anticoagulation
Cisapride	Ventricular arrhythmias[a]
Clarithromycin	Increased APV levels 18%—usual doses
Food	High-fat meal decreases APV absorption 20%; avoid high-fat meal
Ergot alkaloids	Increased ergotamine levels[a]
Ketoconazole	Increase APV levels 31%, ketoconazole levels increased 44%—dose implications unclear
Lovastatin	Increased risk of myopathy[a]
Midazolam	Increased midazolam levels[a]
Pimozide	Pimozide levels increased[a]
Rifabutin	Decreases APV AUC 15% and rifabutin AUC increased 200%—use APV standard dose + rifabutin 150 mg qd
Rifampin	Decreases APV AUC 80%[a]
St John's wort	Decreased amprenavir levels[a]
Simvastatin	Increased rates of myopathy[a]
Sildenafil	Increased sildenafil levels—do not exceed 25 mg/48 hr
Terfenadine	Ventricular arrhythmias[a]
Triazolam	Increased triazolam levels[a]
Antiretrovirals	
Efavirenz	EFV increases 15%, APV levels decrease 24%—EFV 600 mg hs + APV 1200 mg tid or APV 1200 mg bid + RTV 200 mg bid + EFV 600 mg hs
Indinavir	IDV levels decrease 38%, APV levels increase 33%—IDV 800 mg tid + APV 800 mg tid
Nelfinavir	NFV levels increase 15%, APV levels increase 1.5×—NFV 750 mg tid + APV 800 mg tid
Fortovase	SQV levels decrease 19%, APV levels decrease 32%—Fortovase 800 mg tid + APV 800 mg tid (limited data)

Table 46. (continued)

Drug	Effect of Interaction
Lopinavir/ritonavir	APV increased, LPV decreased but data are variable—LPV/r 400/100 mg bid or 533/133 mg bid + APV 750 mg bid
Nevirapine	No data
Delavirdine	DLV decrease 60%, AMP increase 25%[a]
Antiretrovirals + FPV	LPV Cmin decrease 61% and FPV levels decrease 69%—consider LPV/r 4 caps bid + FPV 1400 mg bid—limited data and poorly tolerated; consider APV

Atazanavir (Inhibitor & substrate for P450 A4; requires gastric acid and prolongs QTc)

Drug	Effect of Interaction
Antacids & buffered meds	Give 2 hr before or after ATV; use Videx EC and separate dosing
Astemizole	Ventricular arrhythmias[a]
Bepridil	Increased bepridil levels[a]
Cisapride	Ventricular arrhythmias[a]
Clarithromycin	AUC clarithromycin increased 94%—use half dose
Calcium channel blocker	Monitor EKG
Carbamapezine	Decreased ATV levels—avoid or use caution
Diltiazem	Diltiazem levels increased 125%—use half dose and monitor EKG
Oral contraceptives	Estradiol AUC increased 48% norestradiol increased 110%—use lowest dose or alternative
Didanosine	Use ddI instead of buffered ddI
Ergotamine	Increased ergotamine levels[a]
Irinotecan	Increased irinotecan levels[a]
Lovastatin	Risk of myopathy[a]
Methadone	Unknown
Midazolan	Increased midazolan levels[a]
Pimozide	Increased pimozide levels[a]
Rifabutin	Increases RBT levels—use 150 mg qod or 150 mg 3x/wk
Rifampin	Reduces ATV levels[a]
Proton pump inhibitors	Reduces ATV bioavailability[a]
Simvastatin	Risk of myopathy[a]
St. John's wort	Decreased ATV levels[a]
Sildenafil	Increased sildenafil levels—do not exceed 25 mg/48 hr
Tenofovir	Decrease ATV AUC 25%—use ATV/r 300/100 mg qd
Terfenadine	Ventricular arrhythermia[a]
Vardenafil	No data—use ≤ 2.5 mg mg/24 hr with ATV and ≤ 2.5 mg/24 hr with ATV/r
Antiretrovirals	
Indinavir	Increased indirect bilirubin[a]
Ritonavir	ATV AUC increased 3.4 x—use ATV/r 300/100 mg qd
Saquinavir	SQV AUC increased 4.5x ATV decreased—consider SQV 1600 mg/ ATV 300/r 100 mg qd
Nelfinavir	No data
Amprenavir	No data

Table 46. (continued)

Drug	Effect of Interaction
Fosamprenavir	No data
Efavirenz	ATV AUC decreased 74%; EFV no change—use EFV 600/ATV 300/r 100 mg qd
Nevirapine	No data
Atovaquone	
AZT	Increased AZT levels (significance is ?)
Food (fat)	Increased absorption—should be taken with meals
Rifampin and rifabutin	Decreased atovaquone levels[a]
Sulfa-trimethoprim	Decreased TMP-SMX levels (slight)
Tetracycline	Decreased atovaquone levels (40%)
Azithromycin	
Coumadin	Increased prothrombin time
Pimozide	Ventricular arrhythmias[a]
Theophylline	Increased theophylline levels
AZT (Retrovir, Zidovudine)	
Amphotericin B	Increased anemia
Atovaquone	Increased AZT levels increase 31%—use standard dose
Cancer chemotherapy (adriamycin, vinblastine, vincristine)	Increased marrow toxicity
Clarithromycin	Decreased AZT absorption, give ≥2 hr apart
d4T (Stavudine)	Pharmacologic antagonism
Dapsone	Increased marrow toxicity
Fluconazole (400 mg/day)	Increased AZT levels
Flucytosine	Increased leukocytosis
Ganciclovir	Increased leukopenia, concurrent use usually contraindicated except with G-CSF[a]
Interferon	Increased leukopenia
Methadone	Increased AZT levels—no dose adjustment
Phenytoin	Decreased phenytoin levels
Probenecid	Increased AZT levels but high frequency of rash
Rifampin/rifabutin	Decreased AZT levels
Valproate	Possible AZT toxicity
Benzodiazepines	
Caffeine	Antagonizes sedative effect
Cimetidine	Increased benzodiazepine toxicity
Erythromycin	Increased benzodiazepine toxicity
Isoniazid	Increased benzodiazepine toxicity
Omeprazole	Increased benzodiazepine toxicity
Rifampin, rifabutin	Decreased benzodiazepine effect
Cidofovir	
Nephrotoxic drugs	Aminoglycosides, amphotericin, foscarnet, IV pentamidine, and nonsteroidal antiinflammatory drugs—avoid concurrent use and provide a 7-day ``washout''

Table 46. (continued)

Drug	Effect of Interaction
Probenecid interactions	Probenecid increases T½ of acyclovir, aminosalicylic acid, barbiturates, beta-lactams, AZT, benzodiazepines, bumetanide, methotrexate, famotidine, furosemide, theophylline
Clarithromycin	
Amprenavir	No significant change in either drug
Atazanavir	Clarithromycin AUC increased 94% with risk of prolonged QTc—use half dose clarithro or azithromycin
Carbamazepine (Tegretol)	Increased carbamazepine levels[a]
Cisapride (Propulsid)	Risk of ventricular arrhythmias[a]
Delavirdine	DLV levels increased 44% and clarithromycin levels increased 100%—dose adjust in renal failure
Disopyramide	Increased disopyramide levels[a]
Efavirenz	EFV levels decreased 39% avoid; use azithromycin for MAC
Ergot Alkaloids	Increased ergot toxicity
Indinavir	Clarithromycin levels increased 50% and IDV levels increased 29%—no dose adjustment
Lopinavir/ritonavir	Increase clarithro levels 77%—reduce clarithro dose 50% if CrCl 30–60 mL/min and 75% if CrCl < 30 mL/min
Nevirapine	NVP levels increased 26%, clarithromycin levels decreased 30%—standard doses and monitor or use azithromycin
Pimozide	Risk of ventricular arrhythmia[a]
Rifabutin	Increased rifabutin levels 56% with possible uveitis; decreased clarithro
Rifampin	Decreased clarithromycin levels[a]
Ritonavir	Increased clarithro levels 77%—reduce clarithro dose 50% if CrCl 30–60 mL/min and 75% if CrCl < 30 mL/min
Saquinavir	Increased levels of saquinavir 77%—use standard dose
Terfenadine (Seldane)	Risk of ventricular arrhythmias[a]
Theophylline	Elevated theophylline levels
Agents that prolong QT interval	Cisapride, terfenadine, atazanavir, fluoroquinolones—risk of ventricular arrhythmias
Clindamycin	
Antiperistaltic agents (Lomotil, loperamide)	Increased risk and severity of *C. difficile* colitis[a]
Dapsone	
Coumadin ddl	Increased hypothrombinemia Decreased levels of dapsone, give ≥2 hr apart[a]
H₂ blockers, antacids, omeprazole	Decreased absorption of dapsone
Primaquine	Increased hemolysis with G-6-PD deficiency
Probenecid	Increased dapsone levels

Table 46. (continued)

Drug	Effect of Interaction
Pyrimethamine	Increased marrow toxicity (monitor CBC)
Rifampin and rifabutin	Decreased levels of dapsone by 7-10×; increase dapsone level or use alternative
Saquinavir	Increased dapsone levels
Trimethoprim	Increased levels of both drugs
Warfarin (Coumadin)	Increased prothrombin time

d4T (Stavudine)

AZT	Pharmacologic antagonism[a]
ddI	Increased lactic acidosis, peripheral neuropathy, and pancreatitis—avoid if possible and contraindicated in pregnancy
ddC	Increased peripheral neuropathy[a]
Agents associated with peripheral neuropathy	Increased frequency and severity of peripheral neuropathy: Cisplatin, dapsone, ddI, ddC, disulfiram, ethionamide, glutethimide, gold, hydralazine, iodoquinol, INH, phenytoin, metronidazole (long term), vincristine
Methadone	D4T AUC decreased 24%—use standard doses of both drugs

ddC (HIVID, zalcitabine, dideoxycytidine)

ddI and d4T	Increased peripheral neuropathy[a]
Agents associated with peripheral neuropathy	Increased frequency and severity of peripheral neuropathy: Cisplatin, dapsone, ddI, ddC, d4T, disulfiram, ethioinamide, glutethimide, gold, hydralazine, INH, iodoquinol, metronidazole, nitrofurantoin, phenytoin, vincristine[a]
Agents associated with pancreatitis	Pentamidine, ddI, d4T, rifampin, alcohol abuse

ddI (Videx, didanosine)

Note: All drugs that require gastric acidity for absorption should be given ≥2 hr before or ≥1 hr after buffered ddl. This does *not* apply to Videx EC (enteric-coated ddl). The following applies only to buffered ddl.

Dapsone	Decreased dapsone absorption, give ≥2 hr before or >1 hr after ddl
Delavirdine	Separate dosing by ≥ 2 hrs
Ganciclovir—oral	Separate dosing by ≥ 2 hrs
Ketoconazole, itraconazole	Separate dosing by ≥ 2 hrs
Indinavir	Separate dosing by ≥ 2 hrs
Quinolones	Separate dosing by ≥ 2 hrs
Ritonavir	Separate dosing by ≥ 2 hrs
Atavanavir	ATV AUC is decreased 87%—could use ddl EC, but this requires ddl EC on empty stomach and ATV on full stomach; alternative is to give ATV 2 hr before or 1 hr after buffered ddl

Table 46. (continued)

Drug	Effect of Interaction
Tenofovir	Increases ddl AUC 28%—reduce ddl dose (buffered or Videx EC) to 250 mg qd
Methadone	Decreased ddl AUC 40%; no effect on methadone levels. Consider ddl dose increase
Agents associated with pancreatitis	Pentamidine, rifampin, alcohol abuse, d4T, hydroxyurea
Agents associated with peripheral neuropathy	Increased frequency and severity of peripheral neuropathy: Cisplatin, dapsone, ddC, d4T, disulfiram, ethionamide, glutethimide, gold, hydralazine, iodoquinol, INH, metronidazole, nitrofurantoin, phenytoin, vincristine

Dronabinol (Marinol)

Alcohol	Increased CNS depression
Amitriptyline, amoxapine, other tricyclic antidepressants	Tachycardia, hypertension, drowsiness
Amphetamines, cocaine, and other sympathomimetic drugs	Increased hypertension and tachycardia
Atropine, scopolamine, and other anticholinergic agents	Tachycardia, drowsiness

Efavirenz (induces and inhibits CYP3A)

Astemizole	Ventricular arrhythmias[a]
Carbamazepine	Decreased levels of EFV
Cisapride	Ventricular arrhythmias[a]
Clarithromycin	Decrease clarithromycin levels 39%[a]; rash in 46%—avoid[a]
Ergot alkaloids	Increased ergot levels[a]
Ethinyl estradiol	Increased levels estradiol by 37%—use alternative method
Methadone	Methadone levels reduced 52% monitor for withdrawal or avoid combination
Midazolam	Increased levels midazolam[a]
Phenobarbital	Decreased levels EFV
Phenytoin	Decreased levels EFV
Rifabutin	Rifabutin levels decreased 35% and EFV levels are unchanged; use rifabutin 450 mg–600 mg/day or 100 mg 2×/wk + EFV 600 mg/day
Rifampin	EFV levels decreased 25%—use EFV 800 mg/d
Statins	May need increase in statin dose
Simvastation	Simvastation AUC decreased 58%
Atorvastation	Atorvastation AUC decreased 43%
Pravastation	Pravastation AUC decreased 40%
Rosuvastation or Fluvastation	May be preferred
Terfenadine	Risk of arrhythmias[a]
Triazolam	Increased triazolam levels[a]
Voriconazole	Decrease voriconazole levels[a]
<u>Antiretrovirals</u>	
Atazanavir	ATV AUC decreased 74%, EFV unchanged—use ATV 300/r 100/EFV 600 mg qd
Fosamprenavir	No significant change for either drug—FPV 700 mg bid, RTV 100 mg bid + EFV 600 mg hs

Table 46. (continued)

Drug	Effect of Interaction
Amprenavir	APV levels decreased 36%, EFV no change—APV 600 mg bid + RTV 100 mg bid + EFV 600 mg qd
Indinavir	IDV levels decreased 31%, IDV shows no change—IDV 1000 mg tid + EFV 600 mg/day or IDV 800 mg bid RTV 200 mg bid + EFV 600 mg hs
Lopinavir/ritonavir	LPV levels decreased 40%, EFV no change—EFV 600 mg hs + LPV/r 533/133 (4 caps) bid
Nelfinavir	NFV increased 20%, EFV unchanged—NFV 1250 mg bid + EFV 600 mg/day
Ritonavir	RTV increased 18%, EFV increased 21%—RTV 500-600 mg bid (depending on tolerance) + EFV 600 mg/day
Saquinavir/ritonavir	SQV unchanged, EFV unchanged—standard doses decreased 12%—contraindicated
Emtricitabine (Emtriva)	None
Enfuvirtude (Fuseon)	None

Erythromycins (inhibit cytochrome P450 enzymes)

Anticoagulants (oral)	Increased hypoprothrombinemia
Carbamazepine	Increased carbamazepine levels
Corticosteroids	Increased effect of methylprednisolone
Cyclosporine	Increased cyclosporine levels (nephrotoxicity)
Digoxin	Increased digitalis levels
Disopyramide	Increased disopyramide toxicity[a]
Ergot alkaloids	Increased ergot toxicity[a]
Felodipine	Increased felodipine levels
Phenytoin	Increased phenytoin levels
Propulsid (cisapride)	Ventricular arrhythmias[a]
Tacrolimus	Increased tacrolimus levels
Terfenadine (Seldane)	Ventricular arrhythmias[a]
Theophylline	Increased theophylline levels
Triazolam	Increased triazolam levels
Valproate	Increased valproate levels
Agents that prolong QT interval—cisapride, terfenadine, quinidine, amiodarone, fluoroquinolones	Ventricular arrhythmias

Erythropoietin (EPO)   None

Ethambutol

Al^{++++}-containing drugs	May decrease absorption

Famciclovir

Cimetidine	Increased penciclovir levels
Digoxin	Increased digoxin levels
Probenecid	Increased penciclovir levels
Theophylline	Increased penciclovir levels

Fenofibrate

Coumadin	Potentiates hypoprothrombinemia

Table 46. (continued)

Drug	Effect of Interaction
Cholestyramine	Bind fenofibrate—take fenofibrate >1 hr before or 4-6 hr after bile acid binding agent
Statins	Increased risk of rhabdomyolysis

Fluconazole (inhibits cytochrome P-450)

Drug	Effect of Interaction
Alprazolam	increased sedation
Atovaquone	Increased atovaquone levels
AZT	Increased AZT AUC 74% due to decreased glucuronidation—monitor for AZT toxicity
Benzodiazepines	Increased benzodiazepine levels
Cisapride	Ventricular arrhythmias[a]
Clarithromycin	Increased clarithromycin levels
Contraceptives	Decreased contraception effect—three cases reported
Cyclosporine	Increased cyclosporine levels
Midazolam	Increased sedation
Nortriptyline	Increased sedation and ventricular arrhythmias
Opiate analgesics	Increased opiate effect
Phenytoin	Increased phenytoin levels
Propulsid (cisapride)	Ventricular arrhythmias[a]
Rifabutin	Increased rifabutin levels 80% with possible uveitis[a]—avoid or use RBT 50 mg/d
Saquinavir	Increased saquinavir levels (advantage)
Sulfonylureas	Increased levels with hypoglycemia
Terfenadine (Seldane)	Ventricular arrhythmias[a]
Warfarin (Coumadin)	Increased prothrombin time

Antiretrovirals: Protear inhibitors and non-nucleoside RT inhibitors—no significant drug interactions

Fluoroquinolones (ciprofloxacin, norfloxacin, ofloxacin, lomefloxacin, enoxacin, levofloxacin, moxifloxacin, gatifloxacin)

Drug	Effect of Interaction
Antacids	Decreased fluoroquinolone absorption with Mg-, Ca-, or Al-containing antacids or sucralfate: Give antacid >2 hr after fluoroquinolone
Anticogulants (oral)	Increased hypoprothrombinemia
Caffeine	Increased caffeine effect; primarily with ciprofloxacin and enoxacin; significance?
Cyclosporine	Possible increased nephrotoxicity
Food (dairy product)	Decreased absorption
Iron	Decreased ciprofloxacin absorption[a]
Nonsteroidal anti-inflammatory agents	Possible seizures and increased epileptogenic potential of theophylline, opiates, tricyclics, and neuroleptics
Probenecid	Increased fluoroquinolone levels
Theophylline	Increased theophylline toxicity, especially ciprofloxacin and enoxacin (seizures, cardiac arrest, respiratory failure caused by theophylline toxicity)[a]
Zinc	Decreased ciprofloxacin absorption
Agents that prolong QT interval—atazanavir, erythromycin, clarithromycin, amiodarone, quinidine, procainamide, cisapride	Ventricular arrhythmias

Table 46. (continued)

Drug	Effect of Interaction
Fluoxetine (Prozac)	
Astemizole	Increased astemizole levels
Digitalis	Increased digitalis levels
Haloperidol	Increased haloperidol levels
MAO inhibitors	Risk of serotonergic syndrome—avoid initiating fluoxetine until ≥14 day after discontinuing MAO inhibitor
Saquinavir	Increased saquinavir levels
Terfenadine (Seldane)	Ventricular arrhythmias[a]
Theophylline	Increased theophylline levels
Tricyclics	Increased tricyclic levels
Warfarin (Coumadin)	Increase prothrombin time
Fosamprenavir	See amprenavir
Foscarnet	
Aminoglycosides	Increased renal toxicity
Amphotericin B	Increased renal toxicity
Imipenem	Increased frequency of seizures (?)
Pentamidine	Increased hypocalcemia and renal toxicity[a]
Ganciclovir and valgancyclovir	
AZT (Retrovir)	Increased leukopenia, concurrent use should be used with caution, may need G-CSF
Imipenem	Increased frequency of seizures (?)
Myelosuppressing drugs: TMP-SMX, AZT, azathrioprine, pyrimethamine, flucytosine, interferon, adriamycin, vinblastine, vincristine	Increased neutropenia
Probenecid	Increased ganciclovir levels
Ganciclovir, oral and valacyclovir	
(see above)	
AZT	Increased neutropenia
ddI	Decreased absorption take ≥2 hr apart
Food	Increased ganciclovir levels—should be taken with meals
Myelosuppressing drugs	See previous note
G-CSF and GM-CSF	
Cancer chemotherapy	Should not be given within 24 hr of chemotherapy
Indinavir (inhibits P-450 3A4 enzymes)	
Anticonvulsants (Carbamazepine phenytoin, phenobarbitol)	Decreased indinavir levels
Astemizole	Increased astemizole levels, cardiac arrhythmias[a]
Cisapride	Increased cisapride levels[a]
Clarithromycin	Clarithromycin in levels increased 50%—no dose adjustment
Didanosine (ddI)	Decreased indinavir absorption, take ≥2 hr apart or use Videx EC
Ergot alkaloids	Increased ergot levels[a]
Estradiol	Estradiol levels increased 24%—no dose adjustment

Table 46. (continued)

Drug	Effect of Interaction
Food	Decreased indinavir levels—take on empty stomach or with light meal without fat
Grapefruit juice	Decreased indinavir levels 26%
Ketoconazole	Increased levels of indinavir; reduce indinavir dose to 600 mg q8h
Lovastatin	Increased lovastatin levels[a]
Methadone	No change in levels
Midazolam (Versed)	Increased midazolam levels[a]
Pimozide	Increased pimozide levels[a]
Rifampin and rifabutin	Decreased indinavir levels and increased levels of rifampin or rifabutin, avoid rifampin; reduce rifabutin to 150 mg/d or 300 mg 3×/wk and increase indinivar dose to 1000 mg tid or use IDV/RTV in standard dose and RBT 150 mg qod or 150 mg 3×/wk
St John's wort	Decreased IDV levels 57%[a]
Simvastatin	Increased simvastatin levels[a]
Sildenafil	Increased levels of sildenafil 340%—do not exceed 25 mg/48 hr
Terfenadine (Seldone)	Increased terfenadine levels with cardiac arrhythmias[a]
Triazolam (Halcion)	Increased triazolam levels[a]
Tadalafil	Increase tadalafil—use 5 mg initially and do not exceed 10 mg/72 hrs.
Vardenafil	Vardenafil increased AUC 16×—limit to 2.5 mg/3 days
Voriconazole	No interaction unless IDV + RTV
Antiretrovirals	
Atazanavir	Both increase indirect bilirubin—avoid[a]
Delavirdine	Increase IDV levels 40%, DLV no effect—IDV 600 mg q8h + DLV 400 mg tid
Efavirenz	IDV decreased 31% EFV no effect—IDV 1000 mg q8h + EFV 600 mg/day or IDV 800 mg bid + RTV 200 mg bid + EFV 600 mg hs
Fosamprenavir	No data
Amprenavir	APV increased 31%, IDV decreased 38%—APV 800 mg tid + IDV 800 mg tid
Lopinavir/ritonavir	LPV—no change, IDV increased 3×—IDV 600 mg or 666 mg bid + LPV/r 400/100 mg bid
Nelfinavir	NFV levels increased 80%, IDV increased 50%—IDV 1200 mg bid + NFV 1250 mg bid
Nevirapine	IDV levels decreased 28% NVP—no effect—IDV 1000 mg tid + NVP standard
Ritonavir	Increases in levels of both drugs—IDV 400 mg bid + RTV 400 mg bid or IDV 800 mg bid + RTV 100–200 mg bid
Saquinavir (Invirase)	Increased SQV levels 4–7×; IDV—no effect but possible antagonism—avoid

Table 46. (continued)

Drug	Effect of Interaction
Interferon	
AZT	Increased marrow suppression
Barbiturates	Increased barbiturate levels
Theophylline	Increased theophylline levels
Isoniazid	
Alcohol	Increased risk of INH hepatitis
	Decreased INH effect in some alcholics
Antacids	Decreased INH levels with Al-containing antacids
Benzodiazepines	Increased effects of benzodiazepines
Carbamazepine	Increased toxicity of both drugs[a]
Cycloserine	Increased CNS toxicity, dizziness, drowsiness
Diazepam	Increased diazepam levels—reduce diazepam dose
Disulfiram	Psychotic episodes, ataxia[a]
Ethionamide	Increased CNS toxicity
Enflurane	Possible nephrotoxocity[a]
Food	Decreased absorption
Ketoconazole or itraconazole	Decreased azole effect[a]
Phenytoin	Increased phenytoin toxicity
Rifampin and rifabutin	Possible increased hepatic toxicity
Theophylline	Increased theophylline levels
Tyramine (foods and fluids rich in tyramine—especially cheese, wine, some fish)	Rare patients get palpitations, sweating, urticaria, headache, and/or vomiting
Warfarin (Coumadin)	Increased hypoprothrombinemia
Itraconazole	
(inhibits cytochrome P-450)	Note: caps require gastric acid and should be taken with food; liquid suspension should be taken on empty stomach and does not require acid
Alprazolam	Increased sedation
Astemizole	Increased astemizole levels[a]
Calcium channel blockers	Increased levels of Ca blocker
Carbamazepine (Tegretol)	Decreased itraconazole levels
Cisapride	Ventricular arrhythmias[a]
Coke and other acidic drinks	Increased absorption of caps
Contraceptives	Decreased contraceptive effect
Cyclosporine	Increased cyclosporine levels
ddI	Decreased itraconazole levels—take ≥2 hr apart or use Videx EC
Digoxin	Increased digoxin levels
Food	Increased itraconazole absorption; give with meal
H₂ antagonists, antacids, omeprazole, sucralfate	Decreased itraconazole levels with caps—does not apply to oral itraconazole solution
Hypoglycemics, oral	Severe hypoglycemia
Indinavir	Increased IDV levels—decrease IDV dose to 600 mg tid
Other PIs	No dose changes
NNRTI	No dose changes
Isoniazid	Decreased itraconazole levels[a]

Table 46. (continued)

Drug	Effect of Interaction
Lovastatin	Increased myopathy risk[a]
Midazolam	Increased midazolam levels[a]
Phenobarbitol	Decreased itraconazole levels[a]
Phenytoin	Decreased itraconazole levels[a]
Cisapride (Propulsid)	Ventricular arrhythmias[a]
Rifampin or rifabutin	Decreased itraconazole levels[a]
Simvastatin	Increased myopathy risk[a]
Terfenadine (Seldane)	Ventricular arrhythmias[a]
Triazolam	Increased triazolam effect[a]
Warfarin (Coumadin)	Increased hypoprothrombinemia

Ketoconazole
(inhibits cytochrome P-450)

Drug	Effect of Interaction
Alcohol	Possible disulfiram-like reaction
Alprazolam	Increased sedation
Amprenavir	APV levels increased 31% and ketoconazole levels decreased 44%—dose implications unclear
Antacids	Decreased ketoconazole levels
Astemizole	Ventricular arrhythmia[a]
Cisapride	Increased cisapride levels, ventricular arrhythmias[a]
Contraceptives	Decreased contraceptive effect
Corticosteroids	Increased methylprednisolone levels
Cyclosporine	Increased cyclosporine toxicity
ddI	Decreased ketoconazole levels—give ≥2 hr apart
Efavirenz	Not studied
Food	Decreased ketoconazole absorption—give ≥2 hr apart
H₂ antagonists, antacids, omeprazole	Decreased ketoconazole levels[a] (use sucralfate or take antacids more than 2 hr before)
Hypoglycemics, oral	Severe hypoglycemia
Indinavir	Increased indinavir levels 70%; reduce indinavir dose to 600 mg q8h
Isoniazid	Decreased ketoconazole levels[a]
Lopinavir	Ketoconazole levels increased 3×—dose implications unclear
Loratadine (Claritin)	Increased levels of loratadine
Midazolam	Increased midazolam levels[a]
Nelfinavir	No dose change
Nevirapine	NVP levels increased 15-30%, ketoconazole levels decreased 63%—avoid[a]
Phenytoin	Altered metabolism of both drugs
Rifampin and rifabutin	Decreased activity of both drugs[a]
Ritonavir	Increase ketoconazole levels 3×; do not exceed 200 mg/day
Saquinavir	Increased saquinavir levels by 150% (advantage)
Terfenadine (Seldane)	Ventricular arrhythmias[a]
Theophylline	Increased theophylline levels
Triazolam	Increased triazolam levels[a]
Warfarin (Coumadin)	Increased hypoprothrombinemia

Table 46. (continued)

Drug	Effect of Interaction
Lamivudine (3TC, Epivir)	
AZT	Resistance to 3TC promotes susceptibility to AZT—advocated combination
Trimethoprim	Increases 3TC levels 40% (implications unclear)
Lopinavir-ritonavir	Inhibits P-450 isoenzymes
Astemizole	Risk of arrhythmias[a]
Atorvastatin	Atorvastatin AUC increased 4.5×—use lowered dose— 10 mg/d or alternative such as provastatin, fluvastatin, or rosuvastatin
Carbamazepine	Decreased LPV levels—monitor closely
Clarithromycin	Clarithro levels increased; reduce clarithro dose in renal failure
Cisapride	Risk of arrhythmias[a]
Ergot derivatives	Increased ergot levels[a]
Ethyl estradiol	Ethyl estradiol AUC decreased 42%—use alternative method
Flecainide	Increased flecainide levels[a]
Ketoconazole	Ketoconazole levels increased 3×—limit to ≤200 mg/d
Lovastatin	Risk of myopathy[a]
Methadone	Methadone AUC decreased 53%; monitor for withdrawal
Midazolam	Risk of arrhythmias[a]
Pravastatin	Statin level increased 33%—use standard doses
Pimozide	Risk of arrhythmias
Phenytoin	Decreased LPV levels[a]
Propafenone	Increased propafenone levels[a]
Phenobarbitol	Decreased LPV levels—monitor
Rifabutin	Rifabutin levels increased 5×—decrease RBT dose to 150 mg 3×/week + standard LPV/r dose
Rifampin	Lopinavir levels decreased[a]
St. John's wort	Decreased LPV levels[a]
Simvastatin	Risk of myopathy[a]
Sildenafil	Do not exceed 25 mg/48 hr
Terfenadine	Risk of arrhythmias[a]
Triazolam	Risk of arrhythmias[a]
<u>Antiretrovirals</u>	
Amprenavir	APV levels increased, LPV no change—APV 750 mg bid + LPV/r 533/133 mg (4 caps) bid
Efavirenz	EFV no change, LPV levels decreased 39%—EFV 600 mg hs + LPV/r 533/133 (4 caps) bid
Indinavir	IDV levels increased 3×, LPV unchanged—IDV 600 mg bid + LPV/r 400/100 mg bid
Nevirapine	NVP unchanged; LPV decreased 55%—NVP standard + LPV/r 533/133 mg bid

Table 46. (continued)

Drug	Effect of Interaction
Saquinavir	SQV increased 3-fold—SQV (Fortovase or Invirase) 1000-mg bid + LPV/r 400/100 mg bid
Nelfinavir	Decreased
Delavirdine	Limited data
Atazanavir	Under study—? ATV 300/r 100/LPV/r 3 caps bid ± RTV 100 mg qd
Fosamprenavir	FPV levels decrease 64% and LPV levels decreased 53%—not recommended
Megestrol	None
Methadone	
ABL	Decreased levels of methadone and ABC—clinical implications unclear
Amprenavir	APV levels decreased 35% and methadone levels decreased—consider alternative PI[a]
AZT	Increased AZT levels 44%—no dose adjustment
Alcohol	Increased CNS depression
ddI	Reduces ddI levels 40–60%; may need ddI dose increase
Dronabinol (Marinol)	Increased CNS depression
Efavirenz	Reduction in methadone levels with opiate withdrawal—use with caution, increase methadone dose, or avoid
Indinavir	No change
Lopinavir	Decreased methadone AUC 53%; monitor for withdrawal
Marijuana	Increased CNS depression
Nelfinavir	Methadone levels decreased; monitor for withdrawal
Nevirapine	Reduces methadone levels 60%—monitor for withdrawal, avoid or increase methadone dose
Phenytoin	Decreased methadone levels—anticipate need to increase methadone dose
Rifabutin	No change
Rifampin	Decrease methadone levels—combination contraindicated[a]
Ritonavir	Reduced methadone levels 36%—no dose change
Saquinavir	Decreased methadone levels—no dose change
Metronidazole	
Alcohol	Disulfiram-like reaction
Barbiturates	Decreased metronidazole effect with phenobarbital
Cimetidine	Possible increased metronidazole levels
Corticosteroids	Decreased metronidazole levels
Disulfiram	Organic brain syndrome[a]; stop disulfiram 2 wk before metronidazole

Table 46. (continued)

Drug	Effect of Interaction
Fluorouracil	Transient neutropenia
Food	Reduces gastric irritation
Lithium	Lithium toxicity
Cisapride (Propulsid)	Ventricular arrhythmias[a]
Terfenadine (Seldane)	Ventricular arrhythmias[a]
Coumadin (Warfarin)	Increased hypoprothrombinemia

Nelfinavir (Viracept) (inhibits CYP 3A4 enzymes)

Drug	Effect of Interaction
Astemizole	Ventricular arrhythmias[a]
Cisapride	Ventricular arrhythmias[a]
Ergot alkaloids	Increased ergot levels[a]
Ethinyl estradiol	Decreased levels; use alternative method of birth control
Food	Increases levels 2–3× —must take with food
Lovastatin	Risk of myopathy[a]
Methadone	Methadone levels decreased but standard doses
Midazolam	Increased midazolam levels[a]
Rifabutin	NFV levels decreased 32%, RBT levels increased 2× —NFV 1000 mg tid RBT 150 mg q d reduction by 50% (150 mg QD); nelfinavir levels reduced 32%—increase NFV dose to 1000 mg tid
Rifampin	Reduces nelfinavir levels 82%—avoid[a]
Simvastatin	Risk of myopathy[a]
St John's wort	Decreased NFV levels[a]
Sildenafil	Increased sildenafil levels—do not exceed 25 mg/48 hr
Terfenadine	Ventricular arrhythmias[a]
Triazolam	Increased levels of triazolam[a]

Antiretroviral drugs

Drug	Effect of Interaction
Amprenavir	NFV levels increased 15%, APV increased 1.5× —NFV 1250 mg bid + APV 800 mg tid or 1200 mg bid (limited data)
Delavirdine	Levels 2× and decreased delavirdine levels 50%—avoid
Efavirenz	NFV levels increase 20% EFV no change—standard doses both drugs
Indinavir	Nelfinavir levels increased 80%, IDV levels increased 50%—IDV 1200 mg bid + NFV 1250 mg bid
Lopinavir/ritonavir	No data
Nevirapine	NFV increase 10%, NVP no effect—standard doses
Ritonavir	Nelfinavir levels increased 1.5×, RTV levels unchanged—RTV 400 mg bid + NFV 500–750 mg bid
Saquinavir	Nelfinavir levels increased 20%; saquinavir levels increased 3× —NFV standard + Fortovase 800 mg tid or 1200 mg bid

Table 46. (continued)

Drug	Effect of Interaction
Nevirapine	Induces cytochrome P-450 enzymes
Methadone	Reduces methadone levels 50% monitor methadone dose
Antiretroviral drugs	
Atazanavir	No data, consider ATV/r 300/100 mg NVP, standard
Amprenavir	No data
Fosamprenavir	No data, consider FPV/r 700/100 mg bid and NVP standard dose
Indinavir	IDV decreased 28%, NVP unchanged, IDV 1000 mg q8h + NVP standard
Lopinavir/ritonavir	LPV decreased 50%, NVP no change—LPV/r 533/133 mg (4 caps) bid + NVP standard dose
Nelfinavir	NFV levels increased 10%, NFV unchanged—standard dose
Ritonavir	RTV decreased 11%, NVP no effect—standard doses
Saquinavir	SQV levels decreased 25%, NVP no effect—not recommended
Nortriptyline	
Adrenergic blockers	Increase adrenergic block
Cimetidine	Increased nortriptyline levels
Clonidine	Increased clonidine level
Fenfluramine	Increased fenfluramine levels
Fluconazole	Increased nortriptyline levels
MAO inhibitors	Increased levels of MAO inhibitors[a]
Quinidine	Increased nortriptyline levels
Nystatin	None
Oxandrolone	
Hypoglycemics, oral	Increased hypoglycemia
Warfarin (Coumadin)	Increased anticoagulation
Paromomycin	None
Pentamidine (IV)	
Aminoglycosides	Increased nephrotoxicity[a]
Amphotericin B	Increased nephrotoxicity[a]
Capreomycin	Increased nephrotoxicity[a]
ddI	Increased risk of pancreatitis
Foscarnet	Increased nephrotoxicity[a]
Pyrazinamide	None
Pyrimethamine	
Antacids	Possible decreased pyrimethamine absorption
Dapsone	Agranulocytosis reported
Ganciclovir	Increased neutropenia
Kaolin	Possible decreased pyrimethamine absorption
Lorazepam	Hepatotoxicity
Phenothiazines	Possible chlorpromazine toxicity
Ribavirin	
AZT	Increased risk of anemia

Table 46. (continued)

Drug	Effect of Interaction
ddI	Increased risk of mitochondrial toxicity with lactic acidosis or pancreatitis[a]

Rifabutin (induces cytochrome P-450 for increased hepatic metabolism; effect is less pronounced compared with that of rifampin; both drugs are also metabolized by cytochrome P-450 3A4 so drugs that inhibit these enzymes prolong the half-life of rifabutin and rifampin); see following section for drug interaction affected by this mechanism
See listing for rifampin

Clarithromycin	Increased rifabutin levels and risk of uveitis[a]
Fluconazole	Increased rifabutin levels and risk of uveitis[a]
Antiretroviral agents	
Ritonavir	Increased rifabutin levels and decreased ritonavir levels—RBT 150 mg qod + RTV standard
RTV boosted PI	PI standard + RBT 150 mg qod or 150 mg 3x/wk
Indinavir	Increased rifabutin levels 2× RBT 150 mg/day or 300 mg 3×/wk + IDV 1000 mg q8h
Saquinavir	Increased rifabutin levels, reduced saquinavir levels; concurrent use is contraindicated[a]
Nelfinavir	Increased rifabutin levels 2× and reduced NFV 32% RBT 150 mg/day or 300 mg 3×/wk + NFV 1000 mg tid
Amprenavir	Rifabutin levels increased 193% and AMP level decreased 15% RBT 150 mg/day or 300 mg 3×/week and APV standard
Efavirenz	Rifabutin levels decreased 32% and EFV levels are unchanged—RBT 450–600 mg/day + EFV standard dose
Delavirdine	Decrease DLV levels 80%—contraindicated[a]
Nevirapine	No change for both drugs—RBT 300 mg/d or 300 mg 3×/wk + NVP 200 mg bid
Ritonavir + saquinavir	SQV levels decrease, RBT levels increase 3×—RTV 150 mg 2–3×/wk
Lopinavir + ritonavir	RBT levels increase 3×, LPV unchanged—LPV/r standard, RBT 150 qod or 3×/wk
Atazanavir	RBT levels increased 2.5× and ATV no change—ATV standard dose; RBT 150 mg qod or 3×/wk

Rifampin (induces cytochrome P-450 hepatic enzymes; also metabolized by cytochrome P-450 enzymes)

Aminosaliciclic acid (PAS)	Decreased effectiveness of rifampin; give in separate doses × 8–12 hr
Antiretroviral agents	Levels of delavirdine, atazanavir, fosamprenavir, amprenavir, indinavir, nelfinavir, lopinavir, and saquinavir are decreased; concurrent use is contraindicated with the exception of efavirenz and saquinavir/ritonavir

Table 46. (continued)

Drug	Effect of Interaction
Atovaquone	Decreased atovaquone levels
Barbiturates	Decreased barbiturate levels
Benzodiazepines	Possible decreased benzodiazepine levels
Beta-adrenergic blockers	Decreased beta-blocker levels
Chloramphenicol	Decreased chloramphenicol levels[a]
Clofibrate	Decreased clofibrate levels
Contraceptives	Decreased contraceptive effect[a]
Corticosteroids	Decreased corticosteroid levels[a]
Ciprofloxacin	Increased RBT levels
Clarithromycin	Increased RBT levels
Cyclosporine	Decreased cyclosporine levels[a]
Dapsone	Decreased dapsone levels
Digitalis	Decreased digitalis levels
Disopyramide	Decreased disopyramide levels[a]
Doxycycline	Decreased doxycycline levels
Erythromycin	Increased RBT levels
Estrogens	Decreased estrogen effect; use alternative method of birth control
Fluconazole	Decreased fluconazole levels; increased RBT levels
Food	Decreased rifampin absorption
Haloperidol	Decreased haloperidol levels
Hypoglycemics	Decreased hypoglycemic effect
Isoniazid	Increased hepatotoxicity
Itraconazole	Increased RBT levels
Ketoconazole	Decreased levels of both drugs[a]; increased RBT levels
Methadone	Methadone withdrawal symptoms[a]
Mexiletine	Decreased antiarrhythmic effect
Nifedipine	Decreased antihypertensive effect
Phenytoin	Decreased phenytoin levels
Progestins	Decreased norethindrone levels
Quinidine	Decreased quinidine levels
Theophylline	Decreased theophylline levels
Trimethoprim	Decreased trimethoprim levels
Triazolam	Decreased triazolam levels
Trimetrexate	Decreased trimetrexate levels
Verapamil	Decreased verapamil levels
Warfarin (coumadin)	Decreased hypoprothrombinemia

Ritonavir (profound inhibition of P-450 cytochromes including 3A and 2D6; this is also the major mechanism of ritonavir metabolism). Drugs that should *not* be co-administered: amiodarone, flecainide, propafenone, quinidine, bepridil (Vascor), astemizole, simvastatin, lovastatin, terfenadine (Seldane), cisapride (Propulsid), midazolam (Versed), triazolam (Halcion), pimozide, St John's wort, voriconazole, and ergot alkaloids

Carbamazepine	Decreased ritonavir levels
Atorvastatin	Atorvastatin levels increased 4.5× with RTV/SQV—use lowest atorvastatin dose or use pravastatin, fluvastatin, or rosuvastatin
Clarithromycin	Increase clarithromycin levels 77%—reduce dose in renal failure
Desipramine	Increased desipramine levels—monitor levels of desipramine

Table 46. (continued)

Drug	Effect of Interaction
Didanosine (ddl)	Reduced ritonavir absorption; take ≥2 hr apart or use Videx EC
Ethinyl estradiol	Ethinyl estradiol levels decreased 40%—use alternative method
Erythromycin	Increased erythromycin levels
Fentanyl	Increased fentanyl levels
Food	Modest increase in ritonavir levels—take with meals
Ketoconazole	Increased ketoconazole levels—do not exceed 200 mg/day
Methadone	Methadone levels decreased 8-10%—no dose adjustment; this applies to SQV/r 1600-2000 mg/100 mg qd regimen also consider dose increase
Antiretrovirals	
Amprenavir	APV levels increase 2.5× RTV unchanged—APV 600 mg bid + RTV 100 mg bid or APV 1200 mg/day + RTV 200 mg qd or APV 1200 mg bid + RTV 200 mg bid + EFV 600 mg hs
Atazanavir	ATV levels increased 2.4×—ATV 300 mg and RTV 100 mg qd
Delavirdine	No data
Efavirenz	Levels RTV increase 18%, EFV levels increase 21%—RTV 500-600 mg bid + EFV 600 mg/day; RTV unchanged
Fosamprenavir	FPV AUC increases 2×—FPV/r 700/100 mg bid or FPV/r 1400/200 mg qd
Indinavir	IDV levels increase 2-5×, RTV unchanged—IDV 400 mg bid + RTV 400 mg bid or IDV 800 mg bid + RTV 100 mg bid
Lopinavir/efavirenz	LPV levels decrease 40%, EFV unchanged—LLV/r 533/133 mg bid + EFV 600 mg/day
Nelfinavir	NFV increase 1.5×, RTV unchanged—NFV 500-750 mg bid + RTV 400 mg bid
Nevirapine	No significant interaction—standard doses of each
Saquinavir	SQV levels increase 20×, RTV unchanged—RTV 400 mg bid + SQV 400 mg bid or RTV 100 mg qd + SQV 1600-2000 mg qd or RTV 100 mg bid + SQV 1000 mg bid
Oral contraceptives	Reduced estradiol levels 40%; use alternative method of contraception
Oxycodone	Increased oxycodone levels
Phenobarbitol	Decreased ritonavir levels
Phenytoin	Decreased ritonavir levels
Rifabutin	Rifabutin levels increase 4×, decrease rifabutin dose to 150 mg qod or 150 mg 3×/wk + RTV standard dose
Rifampin	RTV levels decrease 35%, use standard doses both drugs

Table 46. (continued)

Drug	Effect of Interaction
Sildenafil	Increased levels of sildenafil with potential for increased side effects—do not exceed 25 mg/48 hr
St John's wort	Decreased levels RTV[a]
Theophylline	Reduced theophylline levels 43%—monitor theophylline levels
Tricyclic antidepressants	Moderate increased tricyclic levels
Voriconazole	Voriconazole AUC decreased 82% with RTV 400 mg bid—avoid combination with full RTV dose but implications for 100-200 mg/d are unclear
Warfarin	Increased anticoagulant effect
Saquinavir	Inhibition of CYP 34A enzyme
Astemizole	Increase levels of both drugs[a]
Carbamazepine	Decreased saquinavir levels
Cisapride	Increased cisapride levels[a]
Clarithromycin	Increased clarithromycin 45%, SQV levels increased 177%—with SQV + RTV use clarithromycin 150 mg 2-3×/wk
Clindamycin	Increased clindamycin levels
Dapsone	Increased dapsone levels
Dexamethasone	Decrease saquinavir levels
Ergot alkaloids	Increased ergot levels[a]
Fluconazole	Increase saquinavir levels
Food	Fat meal improves bioavailability
Grapefruit juice	Increases saquinavir levels
Ketoconazole	Increase saquinavir levels 3× (advantage) but may increase GI toxicity
Lovastatin	Risk of myopathy[a]
Midazolam	Increased midazolam levels[a]
Phenobarbital	Decreased saquinavir levels
Phenytoin	Decreased saquinavir levels
Antiretrovirals	
Amprenavir	APV levels decrease 32%, SQV decrease 19%—Fortovase 800 mg tid + APV 800 mg tid
Delavirdine	SQV levels increase 5×, DLV no effect—Fortovase 800 mg tid + DLV standard dose
Efavirenz	SQV levels decrease 62%, EFV decrease 12%—combination not recommended
Indinavir	IDV unchanged, SQV increased 4-7×—data inadequate
Lopinavir/ritonavir	LPV levels unchanged, SQV levels increased 3.5×—Fortovase 800 mg bid + LPV/r 400/100 mg bid
Nelfinavir	NFV levels increase 20%, SQV levels increase 3-5×—NFV standard dose, Fortovase 800 mg tid or 1200 mg bid
Nevirapine	SQV levels decreased 25%, NVP no effect—no data

Table 46. (continued)

Drug	Effect of Interaction
Ritonavir	SQV levels increase 20×, RTV no change—SQV (Invirase or Fortovase) 400 mg bid + RTV 400 bid or SQV 1600 mg qd + RTV 100 mg qd or SQV 1000 mg bid + RTV 100 mg bid
Rifabutin	Decreased saquinavir levels by 40%[a], with SQV/RTV use RBT 150 mg qod or 3×/wk
Rifampin	Decreased saquinavir levels by 80%[a] with SQV/RTV use rifampin 600 mg/d or 600 mg 3×/wk
Sildenafil	Increased sildenafil levels—do not exceed 25 mg/48 hr
Simvastatin	Risk of myopathy[a]
St John's wort	Decreased SQV levels[a]
Terfenadine (Seldane)	Increased terfenadine levels with possible ventricular arrhythmias[a]
Triazolam	Increased triazolam levels[a]
Vardenafil	Start with 2.5 mg dose and do not exceed 2.5 mg/72 hr

Serostim (growth hormone)—drug interactions have not been studied

Tenofovir

Atazanavir	ATV AUC decreased 25%—use ATV/r 300/100 mg qd
Didanosine	ddI levels increased 40-60%—use Videx EC 250 mg
Ganciclovir, valganciclovir & cidofovir	Compete with TDF or tubular secretion—monitor for nephrotoxicity
Nephrotoxic drugs	Monitor renal function to adjust TDF dose

Trimethoprim-sulfamethoxazole

Amantadine	Amantadine toxicity with delirium
Ganciclovir	Increased neutropenia
Mercaptopurine	Decreased mercaptopurine levels[a]
Methotrexate	Megaloblastic anemia[a]
Phenytoin	Increased phenytoin levels[a]
Procainamide	Increased procainamide levels
Warfarin (coumadin)	Increased hypoprothrombinemia

Trimetrexate

Acetaminophen	Increased trimetrexate levels
AZT	Increased bone marrow suppression
Cimetidine	Increased trimetrexate levels
Erythromycin	Increased trimetrexate levels
Fluconazole	Increased trimetrexate levels
Ketoconazole	Increased trimetrexate levels
Rifampin, rifabutin	Decreased trimetrexate levels

Vancomycin

Aminoglycosides	Increased nephrotoxicity and possible increased ototoxicity[a]

Table 46. (continued)

Drug	Effect of Interaction
Amphotericin B	Increased nephrotoxicity
Cisplatin	Increased nephrotoxicity
Digoxin	Decreased digoxin levels
Voriconazole	
Alprazolam	Increase alprazolam levels—reduce dose
Astemizole	Increased risk of arrhythmias[a]
Carbamazepine	Decrease voriconazole levels[a]
Cisapride	Increased risk of arrhythmias[a]
Coumadin	Increase prothrombin time-monitor
Calcium channel blockers	Increased level of Felodipine–consider dose decrease
Cyclosporine	Increase cyclosporin level—use half dose cyclosporine dose and monitor levels
Efavirenz	Voriconazole level decreased 77% and EFV level increased 44%[a]
Ergot	Ergot levels increased[a]
Glipizide/glyburide	Increased level sulfonyurea—monitor glucose
Midzolam	Increase midzolam level—monitor
Omeprazole	Omeprazole level increases 2×—use half dose
Pimozide	Increase pimozide level[a]
Phenytoin	Decrease voriconazole level increase voriconazole dose to 900 mg bid or 5 mg/kg bid and monitor phenytoin level
Phenobarbitol	Decrease voriconazole levels[a]
Quinidine	Increased quinidine level[a]
Rifabutin	Decrease voriconazole levels[a]
Rifampin	Decrease voriconazole levels[a]
Ritonavir	Voriconazole AUC decreased 82% with RTV 400 mg bid. This dose is contraindicated for concurrent use but implications for ''baby dose'' RTV are not known
Statins	Anticipate increase in statin levels, consider reduced statin dose
Tacrolimus	Increase tacrolimus levels 2×; use 1/3 dose tacrolimus and monitor levels
Tolbutamide	Increased tolbutamide levels—monitor blood glucose
Terfenadine	Risk of arrhythmias[a]
Triazolam	Increased triazolam levels—reduce dose
Vincristine/vinblastine	Increased levels of vinca alkaloids—use reduced dose

[a] Concurrent use should be avoided if possible.

Table 47. Financial Assistance Programs

Drug	Program	Contact
Abacavir (Ziagen)	Patient assistance	800-722-9294
Acyclovir (Zovirax)	Patient assistance[a]	800-722-9294
Amprenavir (Agenerase)	Patient assistance	800-722-9294
Atazanavir	Patient assistance	800-272-4878
Atovaquone (Mepron)	Patient assistance[a]	800-722-9294
Azithromycin (Zithromax)	Patient assistance[a]	800-207-8990
AZT (Retrovir)	Patient assistance[a]	800-722-9294
Cidofovir (Vistide)	Patient assistance[a]	800-226-2056
Ciprofloxacin (Cipro)	Patient assistance[a]	800-998-9180
Clarithromycin (Biaxin)	Patient assistance[a]	800-659-9050
Clindamycin	Patient assistance[a]	800-242-7014
Delavirdine (Rescriptor)	Patient assistance[a]	888-777-6637
D4T (stavudine, Zerit)	Patient assistance[a]	800-272-4878
ddI (Videx) (didanosine)	Patient assistance[a]	800-272-4878
ddC (Hivid) (Zalcitabine)	Patient assistance[a]	800-282-7780
Efavirenz (Sustiva)	Patient assistance	800-272-4878
Emtricitabine	Patient assistance	800-445-3235
EPO (Procrit)	Patient assistance[a]	800-553-3851
Ethambutol	Patient assistance	800-859-8586
Fluconazole (Diflucan)	Patient assistance[a]	800-207-8990
Fosamprenavir	Patient assistance	800-722-9294
Foscarnet (Foscavir)	Patient assistance[a]	800-488-3247
Ganciclovir (IV and oral)	Patient assistance[a]	800-282-7780
G-CSF (Neupogen)	Patient assistance[a]	
GM-CSF (Leukine)	Patient assistance[a]	800-272-9376
Growth Hormone (Serostin)	Patient assistance	888-628-6673
Indinavir	Patient assistance[a]	800-850-3430
Interferon		
Roferon	Patient assistance[a]	800-443-6676
Intron	Product information and Patient assistance[a]	800-521-7157
Itraconazole (Sporonox)	Patient assistance[a]	800-652-6227
Ketoconazole (Nizoral)	Patient assistance[a]	800-652-6227
Lamivudine (3TC)	Patient assistance[a]	800-722-9294
Lopinavir	Patient assistance[a]	800-659-9050
Megestrol (Megace)	Patient assistance[a]	800-272-4878
Nelfinavir (Viracept)	Patient assistance[a]	800-777-6637
Nevirapine	Patient assistance[a]	800-556-8317
Nystatin	Patient assistance[a]	800-272-4878

Table 47. (continued)

Drug	Program	Contact
Oxandrolone (Oxandrin)	Patient assistance[a]	866-692-6374
Pegylated Interferon (Peg-Intron)	Patient assistance	800-521-7157
Pegasys	Patient assistance	877-734-2797
Pentamidine (Pentam)	Patient assistance[a]	888-391-6300
Pyrimethamine	Patient assistance[a]	800-722-9294
Rifabutin	Patient assistance[a]	800-242-7014
Ritonavir (Norvir)	Patient assistance[a]	800-659-9050
Saquinavir (Invirase, Fortovase)	Patient assistance[a]	800-282-7780
Serostim (growth hormone)	Patient assistance and annual $36,000 cap	888-628-6673
Tenofovir (Viread)	Patient assistance[a]	800-445-3235
Thalidomide	Availability from STEPS (Celgene)	888-423-5436
Trizivir	Patient information	800-722-9294
Zidovudine (AZT, Retrovir)	Patient assistance[a]	800-722-9294

[a] Usual requirements are lack of prescription drug insurance (including state plans and Ryan White funds) usually accompanied with income/asset criteria.

10—Major Complications of HIV Infection

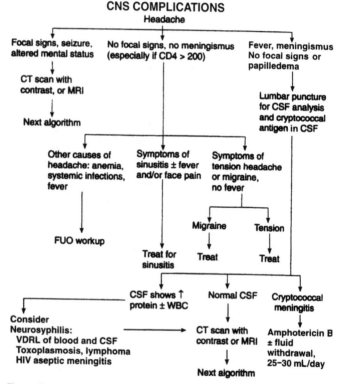

Figure 3. Headache. CT, computed tomography; MRI, magnetic resonance imaging; CSF, cerebrospinal fluid; FUO, fever of unknown origin; WBC, white blood cell count; VDRL, venereal disease research laboratory.

Table 48. Central Nervous System Infection: Differential Diagnosis

Agent	Course	Frequency Setting	Typical Findings	Diagnosis
Toxoplasmosis	Acute	Common: 3–10% of all AIDS patients; 20–35% of AIDS patients with CD4 <100 plus positive serology without prophylaxis	*Mental status*—reduced; *temp:* fever; *scar:* ring-enhanced lesions with mass effect and usually multiple lesions widely distributed; *CSF:* increased protein and 0–40 monos; nl 25%	Typical clinical and scan findings; Response to empiric treatment with clinical improvement in ≤1 wk or scan improvement in 2 wk; IgG serology positive in 85–95%
Lymphoma	Typically subacute	3% of all AIDS patients CD4 <100	*Mental status*—variable; *temp:* afebrile; *scar:* solid-enhanced lesions with mass effect; *location:* periventricular, multiple in 60%; *CSF:* increased protein and 0–100 monos; nl 40%	Typical clinical and scan findings ± failure to respond to empiric treatment of toxoplasmosis; PCR for Epstein-Barr virus in CSF
PML	Subacute	1–3% of all AIDS patients, CD4 <200	*Mental status*—alert; *temp:* afebrile; *scar:* punctate, nonenhanced discrete multifocal lesions without mass effect; *location:* subcortical white matter; *CSF:* normal	Typical clinical and scan findings; stereotactic biopsy-antibody to SV40; characteristic inclusions in oligodendrocytes; PCR for JC virus (20% false negative)
Cryptococcal	Acute, subacute, or chronic	Common: 8–12% of all AIDS patients; CD4 <100; median—20	*Mental status*—alert; *temp:* fever; *scar:* no focal lesions; *location:* basal ganglia; *CSF:* increase protein, 0–100 monos, decreased glucose, nl in 20%	CSF: cryptococcal antigen (>99%) and positive culture; blood: cryptococcal antigen positive in >95% with meningitis

Table 48. (continued)

Agent	Course	Frequency Setting	Typical Findings	Diagnosis
AIDS dementia complex (ADC)	Subacute or chronic	20–30% of all AIDS patients; CD4 <100	*Mental status*—alert; *temp:* afebrile; *scan:* atrophy and ill-defined changes of deep white matter; *location:* deep white matter; CSF: increased protein and 5–10 monos; nl 40%	Neuropsychiatric tests (HIV Dementia Scale) show subcortical dementia combined with typical scan; mini-mental is insensitive
CMV encephalitis	Acute/subacute	1–2% of all AIDS patients; CD4 <50	*Mental status*—delirious, lethargy; *temp:* fever; no focal signs; *scan:* periventricular infection; CSF: increased protein, decreased glucose, 10–1000 monos	CSF: Cultures negative, PCR usually positive; typical clinic setting and scan: empiric anti-CMV therapy
Neurosyphilis	Asymptomatic Meningeal Tabes dorsalis General paresis Meningovascular Ocular	0.5%; any stage	Variable with stage CSF: increased protein, 5–100 monos ± VDRL	Blood VDRL and FTA-ABS positive + typical CSF changes; CSF VDRL + in 65%; specificity—100%
Tuberculosis	Chronic	0.5–1%; CD4 <350	*Mental status*—reduced; *temp:* fever; *scan:* intracerebral enhancing lesions in 50–70%; CSF: increased protein, 5–2000 monos; decreased glucose, nl 5–10%	Chest x-ray; culture positive from any site; CSF culture positive in 20%; PCR has high yield. PPD variable

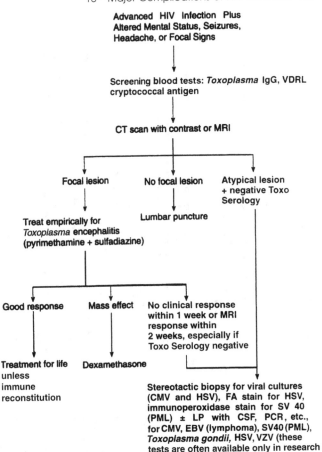

Figure 4. CNS evaluation. CT, computed tomography; MRI, magnetic resonance imaging; FA, fluorescent antibody; PML, polymorphonuclear leukocyte.

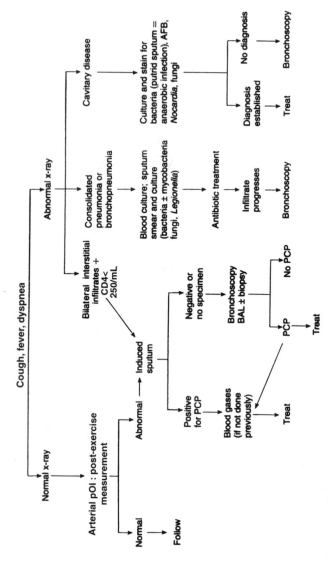

Figure 5. Pulmonary complications.

Table 49. Pulmonary Infection: Differential Diagnosis

Agent	Course[a]	Frequency Setting	Typical Findings	Diagnosis[b]
Bacteria				
S. pneumoniae	Acute	Common, all stages HIV infection	Lobar or bronchopneumonia ± pleural effusion	Sputum GS, quellung, culture, urinary antigen, blood culture
H. influenzae	Acute	Moderately common; all stages HIV infection	Bronchopneumonia	Sputum GS and culture
Gram-negative bacilli	Acute	Uncommon, except with nosocomial infection, neutropenia, chronic antibiotic exposure, structural disease or late stage disease (especially P. aeruginosa)	Lobar or bronchopneumonia, cavity	Sputum GS and culture, Blood culture
Legionella[c]	Acute	Unusual except in epidemic and endemic areas	Bronchopneumonia multiple noncontiguous segments	Legionella urinary antigen ± culture on selective media
S. aureus	Acute	Uncommon except with influenza or tricuspid valve endocarditis with septic emboli in drug abusers	Bronchopneumonia or multiple nodules ± cavitation	Blood cultures (endocarditis), sputum, GS, and culture
Nocardia[c]	Chronic or asymptomatic	Uncommon; late stage HIV	Nodule or cavity	Sputum or FOB; GS, modified AFB stain and culture
Mycobacteria tuberculosis (MTB)[c]	Chronic, subacute, or asymptomatic	Risk with HIV is ↑ 100-fold; all stages—mean CD4 is 200–300/mm³; extrapulmonary TB and atypical pulmonary TB common presentation with CD4 <100	Variable: Focal infiltrates, reticular, cavity disease, hilar adenopathy, lower and middle lobe involvement common, pleural effusion	Sputum AFB stain and culture; induced sputum or bronchoscopy

Table 49. (continued)

Agent	Course[a]	Frequency Setting	Typical Findings	Diagnosis[b]
M. avium complex (MAC)	Chronic	Infrequent; CD4 <50; disseminated MAC with bacteremia and no pulmonary involvement is far more common	Variable	Recovery in sputum or FOB: Must distinguish from MTB (DNA or radiometric culture technique); MA may colonize airways without causing pulmonary disease
M. kansasii	Chronic or asymptomatic	Uncommon: Late-stage HIV, CD4 <50	Cavity disease, nodule, cyst, infiltrate	Recovery in sputum or FOB
Fungi				
Pneumocystis carinii[c]	Subacute or chronic	Very common in late stages of HIV infection (CD4 <200; median CD4 130 without prophylaxis, 30 with prophylaxis)	Interstitial infiltrates; negative x-ray in 10–30%; also has ↑LDH (90%), ↓ pO₂ (95%), ↓ pulse oximetry, ↓ diffusing capacity	Cytopath of induced sputum or FOB, yield with induced sputum 40–80% (average 60%) and depends on quality assurance, yield with FOB BAL: >95%
Cryptococcus neoformans	Chronic, subacute, or asymptomatic	Moderately common: Advanced HIV infection; median CD4 is 50; 80% have cryptococcal meningitis	Nodule, cavity, diffuse, or nodular infiltrates	Sputum or FOB stain and culture, serum usually shows cryptococcal antigen, LP indicated
Histoplasma capsulatum[c]	Chronic or subacute	Uncommon outside endemic area, usually advanced HIV infection with disseminated histoplasmosis—median CD4 is 50	Diffuse or nodular infiltrates, nodule, focal infiltrate, cavity, hilar adenopathy	Sputum or FOB stain and culture; serum and/or urine antigen assay positive in 80–90%; highest yield with culture: Marrow

Coccidioides immitis[c]	Chronic or subacute	Uncommon outside endemic area, median CD4 is 50	Diffuse or nodular infiltrates, focal infiltrate, cavity, hilar adenopathy	Sputum or FOB stain and culture, serology
Candida	Chronic or subacute	Common isolate, rare cause of pulmonary disease, median CD4 is 50	Bronchitis, rare cause of pulmonary infiltrate	Recovery in sputum or analysis of respiratory specimens is meaningless, should have histological evidence of invasion on biopsy
Aspergillus	Acute or subacute	Up to 4% of patients with advanced HIV infection, corticosteroids and neutropenia (ANC <500/mm³)	Focal infiltrate, cavity often pleural-based: changes on CT scan or x-ray are often typical	Sputum stain and culture: False-positive and false-negative cultures common; most reliable are positive stain in typical setting with characteristic scan or x-ray or biopsy evidence of tissue invasion
Virus CMV	Subacute or chronic	Common isolate, rare cause of pulmonary disease; advanced HIV infection with median CD4 <20	Interstitial infiltrates	Yield of CMV by cytopath or culture with FOB is 20–50%; diagnosis of CMV pneumonitis requires CMV by biopsy or CMV plus progressive disease *and* no alternative pathogen
Influenza[c]	Acute	Influenza is common; influenza pneumonia is rare; any stage of HIV infection frequency but severity is greater compared to patients without HIV infection	URI, pharyngitis, bronchitis—most common. Bronchopneumonia or interstitial infiltrates are rare except with bacterial superinfection	Culture or rapid stain for influenza virus with respiratory secretions; physician diagnosis based on clinical symptoms in a flu epidemic has a sensitivity of 70%

Table 49. (continued)

Agent	Course[a]	Frequency Setting	Typical Findings	Diagnosis[b]
Miscellaneous Kaposi's sarcoma	Chronic or asymptomatic	Moderately common in patients with cutaneous KS	Interstitial, alveolar, or nodular infiltrates; hilar adenopathy; pleural effusions; gallium scan usually negative	FOB: Characteristic endobronchial lesion often seen; yield with FOB biopsy of parenchymal lesion is only 10–30%
Lymphoma	Chronic or asymptomatic	Uncommon but may be presenting site	Interstitial, alveolar, or nodular infiltrates; cavity, hilar adenopathy, pleural effusions	FOB: Yield with transbronchial or lymph node biopsy is variable; may need transmediastinal or open lung biopsy or alternative site usually required
Lymphocytic interstitial pneumonia (LIP)	Chronic or subacute	Uncommon in adults CD4 often >200	Diffuse reticular infiltrates, focal infiltrate	FOB: Yield with biopsy is 30–50%; open lung biopsy often required

[a] Course: Acute—symptoms evolve over days; subacute—symptoms evolve over 2–6 wk; chronic—symptoms evolve over >4 wk.
[b] Diagnosis: Expectorated sputum for bacterial culture should have cytological screening to show predominance of PMN; Gram stain (GS) and quellung (if Gram stain suggest S. pneumoniae). Induced sputum is usually reserved for patients with nonproductive cough and suspected PCP or M. tuberculosis. Fiberoptic bronchoscopy (FOB) assumes bronchoveolar (avage specimen (BAL) ± touch preps, bronchial washings, bronchial brush, or transbronchial biopsy. Detection of fungi includes stains (KOH and/or Gomori's methenamine-silver stain) and culture (Sabouraud's agar); Candida spp. grow on conventional bacteria media. Detection of viruses includes cytopathology for inclusions (herpes viruses—CMV, HSV, VZV); FA for HSV and rapid tests for influenza (see Med Lett 1999;41:121).
[c] Detection of these organisms in respiratory secretions is essentially diagnostic of disease. Other organisms may be contaminants, colonizing mucosal surfaces or commensals.

Gastrointestinal Complications

Table 50. Oral Lesions: Differential Diagnosis

Condition	Clinical Features	Diagnosis
Candidiasis (thrush)	White plaques on inflammed base; CD4 count <300 ± antibiotics	Usually a clinical diagnosis; KOH or Gram stain shows yeast and pseudomycelia
Oral hairy leukoplakia	White hairlike projections usually on lateral surface of tongue; CD4 count <300	Usually a clinical diagnosis and often mistaken for thrush. Biopsy shows hairlike projections with EBV by FA stain
Herpes simplex	Small painful vesicles on inflamed base, especially palate or gingiva; any CD4 count but chronic and severe with <100	Usually a clinical diagnosis in patient with history of "cold sores." Smear will show multinucleate giant cells with HSV by FA stain and culture
Aphthous ulcers	Crops of painful ulcers on mucosal surface; any CD4 count	Negative evaluation for HSV, CMV, VZV
Kaposi's sarcoma	Purple or black nodules usually on palate or gingiva; CD4 count <300	Clinical appearance. Biopsy may confirm diagnosis

Table 51. Dysphagia/Odynophagia: Differential Diagnosis

Condition	Clinical Features	Diagnosis
Candida esophagitis	Accounts for 50–70%. Usually has thrush, diffuse esophageal pain, afebrile, CD4 count <100	Usually a presumed diagnosis with odynophagia and thrush Endoscopy—white plaques, brushing or histology shows yeast; culture should not be done except to test for *Candida* azole resistance
CMV	Accounts for 10–20%. Pain is focal and severe, fever is common, CD4 count <100	Biopsy required for treatment Endoscopy shows one or multiple ulcers; biopsy shows CMV inclusions; culture not recommended
Herpes simplex	Accounts for 2–5%. Usually has oral ulcers, focal pain, fever uncommon, CD4 count <100	Endoscopy shows small confluent ulcers; biopsy shows HSV inclusions, positive FA stain, and culture
Idiopathic (aphthous ulcers)	Accounts for 10–20%. Focal pain, afebrile, CD4 count variable	Negative evaluation for pathogens Endoscopy—appears like CMV

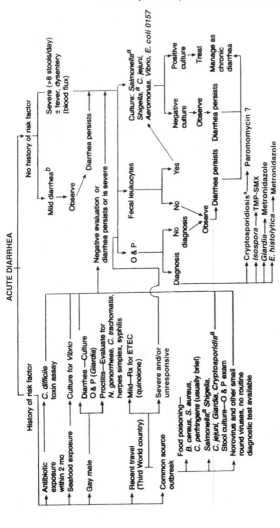

Figure 6.   Acute diarrhea with or without fever. [a] Pathogens considered more frequent and/or severe in patients with advanced HIV infection. [b] Most diarrhea is due to medications (especially ddI, LPV/r, NFV, Fortovase), anxiety, irritable bowel syndrome, or untreatable viral agents (Norwalk agent, other small round viruses, etc.); factors that increase the likelihood of a treatable pathogen are severity of diarrhea, presence of fever, and fecal leukocytes and/or blood.

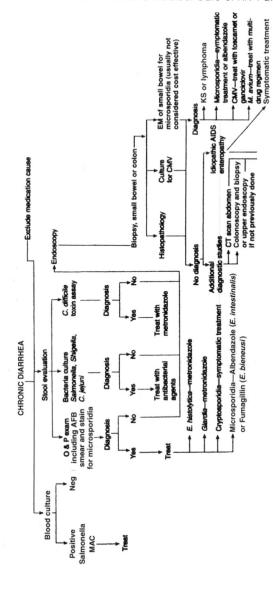

Figure 7. Chronic diarrhea with or without wasting with advanced HIV infection. ^a Lower endoscopy is appropriate as initial endoscopy procedure if there is evidence of colonic disease by symptoms (cramps, dysentery, tenesmus), fecal white blood cells, fecal blood, or CT scan. Upper endoscopy is preferred if there is large volume of diarrhea without fever or cramps and negative fecal WBC exam.

Table 52. Diarrhea: Differential Diagnosis

Agent	Course[a]	Frequency/Setting	Typical Findings	Diagnosis[b]
Bacteria				
Salmonella	Acute or subacute	5–15% of acute diarrheas; any stage of HIV	Enteric fever or gastroenteritis	Blood and stool culture; fecal WBC variable
Shigella	Acute	1–3% of acute diarrheas; any CD4 count	Dysentery (blood and mucus); fever common; colitis	Stool culture; fecal WBC usually present
C. jejuni	Acute	4–8% of acute diarrheas; any CD4 cell count	Stools watery or dysenteric; fever variable; colitis	Stool culture; fecal WBC often present
C. difficile	Acute or chronic	10–15% of acute diarrheas; virtually always with antibiotic exposure, especially clindamycin, ampicillin, or cephalosporins	Stools watery; fever and leukocytosis common; colitis; serum albumin usually low	C. difficile toxin assay; fecal WBC variable
Small bowel overgrowth	Chronic	Frequency unknown	Stools watery; no fever malabsorption	Small bowel aspirate for quantitative culture and/or hydrogen breath test; fecal WBC negative
Mycobacteria				
M. avium	Chronic	10–20% of chronic diarrheas; CD4 <50	Watery diarrhea; enteritis	Most patients have MAC bacteremia with fever Small bowel biopsy with AFB stain ± culture; fever, abdominal pain
Parasites				
Cryptosporidium	Acute or chronic	20–30% of chronic diarrheas CD4 <200	Stools watery, up to 20 L/d 2/3 afebrile, enteritis	Stool AFB or DFA stain or DFA; shows typical oocytes; fecal WBC negative
Isospora	Chronic	1–2% of chronic diarrheas; CD4 <100	Stools watery, fever uncommon, enteritis	Stool AFB smear, fecal WBC negative

Table 52. (continued)

Agent	Course[a]	Frequency/Setting	Typical Findings	Diagnosis[b]
Microsporidia	Chronic	15–20% of chronic diarrheas; CD4 <50	Stools watery, fever uncommon, enteritis	Trichrome stain or other special stain of stool to detect microsporidia
Giardia	Chronic	1–2% of chronic diarrheas; more common in gay men and travelers; any CD4 count	Watery diarrhea ± malabsorption; no fever; symptoms include bloating, flatulence; enteritis	Stool O & P exam; Giardia antigen assay
E. histolytica	Chronic or subacute	1–2% of chronic diarrheas more common in gay men and travelers; any CD4 count	Asymptomatic carriage common, especially in gay men; symptoms include bloody stools and fever; colitis	Stool O & P exam; stool shows RBCs; ability of techs to find trophs highly variable—suggest three stool specimens; endoscopy with scraping or biopsy; serology—IFA titer ↑
Cyclospora cayetanensis	Chronic	<1 of chronic diarrheas	Watery diarrhea	AFB on stool shows circular organisms larger than Cryptosporidium
Viruses CMV	Chronic or subacute	10–40% of chronic diarrheas; CD4 count <50	Enteritis or colitis; represents disseminated CMV; fever, pain; may cause colonic perforation, acute bleed	Intestinal biopsy to show CMV inclusions ± culture; CMV sometimes seen in absence of inflammation or symptoms

	Course	Frequency	Clinical Features	Diagnosis
Enteric viruses	Acute or chronic	15–30% of acute diarrheas; any CD4 count	Enteritis: watery diarrhea	Major agents cannot be detected by clinical labs—astrovirus, adenoviruses, caliciviruses, picobirnavirus
Idiopathic	Chronic	20–30% of chronic diarrheas	Watery diarrhea, small intestinal biopsy shows ↓ villus; crypt ratio without ↑ intraepithelial lymphocytes	Diagnosis based on typical histological changes and negative studies for microbial cause

[a] Course: Chronic indicates diarrhea for most days during ≥1 mo.
[b] Diagnosis: 1) Stool culture in most labs includes selective media for *Shigella, Salmonella,* and *C. jejuni* ± *E. coli* 0157, *Aeromonas, Plesiomonas, Yersina,* and *Vibrios.* 2) Preferred test for *C. difficile* is the EIA or tissue culture assay. 3) O & P exam should be done in fresh stool or stool fixed with polyvinyl alcohol. 4) Modified AFB stain detects *Cryptosporidia, Isospora, Cyclospora,* and *M. avium.* 5) Fecal WBC exam distinguishes "inflammatory" and "secretory" diarrheas: A positive result specifically suggests CMV *Salmonella, Shigella, C. jejuni, C. difficile, Yersina, Aeromonas,* or *Vibrio parahemolyticus.* 6) Serology is useful primarily for *E. histolytica* using IFA, which is increased in 85% with amebic colitis. Endoscopy includes protoscopy, sigmoidoscopy, colonoscopy, and small bowel endoscopy; these are in ascending order of cost and diagnostic utility for unselected AIDS patients and diarrhea. Proctoscopy is preferred for patients with proctitis (usually caused by STDs, including *N. gonorrhoeae, Chlamydia trachomatis,* herpes simplex, and syphilis); small bowel endoscopy with duodenal biopsy has highest yield in patients with "noninflammatory" chronic diarrhea in late stages of HIV infections; colonoscopy or sigmoidoscopy is preferred in patients with evidence of colitis (i.e., pain, fever, tenesmus, bloody stools, and/or fecal leukocytes).

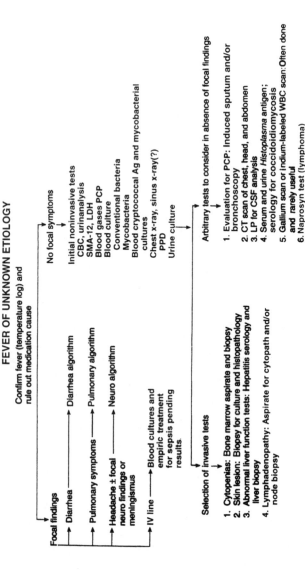

Figure 8. Fever of unknown etiology. Most common causes are TB, PCP, disseminated MAC, lymphoma, and/or drug fever.

Table 53. Dermatologic Complications: Differential Diagnosis

Condition	Presentation	Diagnosis
Adverse drug reaction	Red, papular, pruritic rash most common. Less common: Urticaria, erythema multiforme, photosensitivity Any CD4 count	Response to drug holiday usually adequate unless severe or unresponsive Association with drugs, especially TMP-SMX, dapsone, nevirapine, delavirdine, or efavirenz
Bacillary angiomatosis	Papules or nodules. Resembles Kaposi's sarcoma CD4 variable, usually <200	Biopsy: Warthin—Starry stain shows *B. henselae* Responds to erythromycin
Cryptococcosis	Nodular, ulcerative, or vesicular lesions may resemble HSV, VZV, or molluscum CD4 <100	Biopsy: Methenamine stain shows yeast
Eosinophilic folliculitis	Pruritic papules and pustules; CD4 <250	Biopsy: Eosinophilic infiltrate in follicular epithelium
Herpes simplex	Vesicles with erythematous base—oral, genital, perirectal, or general cutaneous Chronicity and severity inversely related to CD4 count	Tzanck preparation showing multinucleate giant cells; FA stain and/or culture for HSV ± sensitivity tests in refractory cases Biopsy
Herpes zoster	Vesicles on erythematous base in dermatomal distribution. Complications are pain, including postherpetic neuralgia, disseminated disease, blindness; any CD4 count	Tzanck preparation shows multinucleate giant cells Distinguish from HSV by culture or FA stain
Kaposi's sarcoma	Firm subcutaneous brown-black or purple nodules, any cutaneous site, especially face, chest, genitals, extremities	Must distinguish from bacillary angiomatosis Biopsy

Table 53. (continued)

Condition	Presentation	Diagnosis
Molluscum contagiosum	Pearly white or flesh-colored papules with central umbilication; most common on face and genitals	Usually clinical appearance EM of scraping of vesicle fluid
Psoriasis	Plaques that are sharply demarcated, especially knees, elbows, scalp, lumbosacral area	Biopsy with histopath may resemble seborrhea or drug eruption
Seborrhea	Erythematous, scaling plaques with indistinct margins, especially scalp, butterfly region of face, ears, hairline, chest, upper back, axilla, groin	Clinical features
S. aureus	Folliculitis ± pruritus, especially trunk, groin, face	Exudate should show typical GPC and grow S. aureus

INDEX

Note: Page numbers followed by *t* refer to tables; page numbers followed by *f* refer to figures.